Transforming Emotions with Chinese Medicine

SUNY series in Chinese Philosophy and Culture

Roger T. Ames, editor

Transforming Emotions with Chinese Medicine

An Ethnographic Account from Contemporary China

YANHUA ZHANG

STATE UNIVERSITY OF NEW YORK PRESS

Published by
STATE UNIVERSITY OF NEW YORK PRESS,
ALBANY

For information, address
State University of New York Press
194 Washington Avenue, Suite 305, Albany, NY 12210-2384

Production by Christine Hamel
Marketing by Michael Campochiaro

Library of Congress Cataloging-in-Publication Data

Zhang, Yanhua.
    Transforming emotions with Chinese medicine : an ethnographic account from contemporary China / Yanhua Zhang.
        p. cm. -- (SUNY series in Chinese philosophy and culture)
    Includes bibliographical references and index.
    ISBN-13: 978-0-7914-6999-6 (hardcover : alk. paper)
    ISBN-13: 978-0-7914-7000-8 (pbk. : alk. paper)
    1. Medical anthropology--China.   2. Medicine, Chinese.   3. Traditional medicine--China.   4. Ethnopsychology--China.   5. Emotions--Social aspects--China.   I. Title.   II. Series.
GN296.5.C6Z53 2007
306.4´610951--dc22

                                                                    2006012941

10   9   8   7   6   5   4   3   2   1

For my parents.

Contents

Tables

Illustrations

Acknowledgments

This book has benefited from the generous assistance and support of many individuals and institutions. The study leading to this book began at the University of Hawaii at Manoa when I was a graduate student. I have had wonderful teachers: Roger Ames, Jack Bilmes, Fred Blake, Nina Etkin, Allen Howard, Thomas Maretzki, Anthony Marsella, Gregory Maskarinec, and Geoffrey White. They have directly and indirectly contributed to the formation of many ideas in this book. I owe special thanks to Fred Blake, the chair of my dissertation committee, whose guidance and encouragement saw me through the arduous process of dissertation writing, and to Roger Ames, who read the manuscript several times and whose critical comments are largely responsible for the improvement of the present book from the original dissertation. Several other people have read the entire or parts of the manuscript at its different stages. John DeFrancis meticulously went over my bilingual transcript of the clinical interaction and offered detailed corrections and suggestions; Judith Farquhar read and commented on an earlier version of the chapter on *zhongyi* clinical classifications; and Louis Bregger at Clemson University proofread the entire manuscript at least twice. My colleague, Joan Bridgwood, helped with the final proofreading of the book. I am thankful for their assistance.

During the long process of the research and writing of this book, I learned a lot from my fellow graduate students and colleagues through conversations and discussions. I benefited from the insights, criticism, and camaraderie of Weirong Cai, Nancy Cooper, Dphrosine Daniggelis, Bingzhong Gao, Melissa Schrift, Chenshan Tian, Yanyin Zhang, Deborah Zvosec, and many others.

My field research benefited greatly from the help and support of many friends and colleagues in Beijing, China. I want to thank my affiliated institution in Beijing, the School of Ethnology and Sociology at Central University for Nationalities, for hospitality and institutional support. I want especially to thank Yang Shengmin and Teng Xing for introducing me to their network of social relations and helping arrange my fieldwork site. I thank all the students and practitioners of Chinese medicine I met and interacted with in Beijing, particularly Wang Xiuzhen and Cao Pei. They generously shared their knowledge and experience of Chinese medicine with me and patiently answered my questions. Director Zhou Shaohua of Xiyuan hospital provided me with the best fieldwork environment I could ever hope for. He was not only the best *zhongyi* teacher to me, but also my most knowledgeable resource in Chinese medicine. I am also deeply grateful to the patients involved in my research for their trust and generosity. My responsibility to protect their anonymity prevents me from naming them individually, but my deepest gratitude goes to them.

My field research was funded by a grant (Grant No. 5668) from the Wenner-Gren Foundation. I would also like to acknowledge the assistance and support from the Center for Chinese Studies at the University of Hawaii at Manoa. The opportunities to work in their various China-related projects and access to their resources facilitated the completion of the original dissertation. For this, I am particularly thankful to Cynthia Ning, the associate director of the Center, and Daniel Tschudi. Course relief provided by the Department of Languages of Clemson University helped speed up the writing of the final version of this book.

My thanks also go to everyone at SUNY press whose hard work helped to turn my manuscript into this book.

My parents supported my professional pursuit in every way they could. They acted as surrogate parents to my daughter for many years while I was away doing my graduate studies in the U.S.; and they housed me while I was doing fieldwork in Beijing.

Cover Calligraphy by Michael M. Chen.

I.

Introduction

This book offers an ethnographic account of emotion-related disorders as they are understood, experienced, and treated in the clinics of Chinese medicine or *zhongyi* 中医 in contemporary China. Central to this enquiry is a *zhongyi* category of illness, *qingzhi bing* 情志病 or *qingzhi lei jibing* 情志类疾病 (emotion-related disorders),[1] attributable to disordered emotions and treatable with ordinary Chinese medical therapies. What needs to be emphasized from the very beginning is that *qingzhi bing* is not a direct translation of the Western psychiatric concept of "emotional disorder" or "mental disorder." Not a strictly defined discrete illness entity in a biomedical sense, the *zhongyi* construct is used somewhat loosely to include a group of illness patterns, originating from "internal damages attributable to excessive emotions" (*qingzhi neishang* 情志内 伤) and marked with certain configurations of physical, emotional, and behavioral symptoms. While to group disorders predominantly involving emotions and thoughts under the heading of *qingzhi* is nothing modern,[2] the meaning of *qingzhi* disorders encountered in today's *zhongyi* clinics reflects ongoing social and political dynamics in contemporary Chinese society and changes in the profession of Chinese medicine itself through decades of the state-sponsored *zhongyi* modernization under the guidance of science. Biomedical terminology and technology are commonly present in contemporary *zhongyi* practices, yet the way in which a *qingzhi* disorder is conceptualized, experienced, diagnosed, and treated remains remarkably "Chinese." It is not "culturally bound," but certainly "permeated with culture."[3]

THEORETICAL ORIENTATIONS

It is quite common for a medical anthropologist to imagine culture as a shared, unified set of beliefs and values that produce, cause, or govern and thus explain illness and health behaviors. The earlier studies of "culture-bound syndromes" exemplifies this approach, in which culture is seen as playing either a "patho-genic" or "pathoplastic" role in the manifestation of syndromes, such as *amok* and *latah* in Southeast Asia.[4] Most cross-cultural studies of psychiatric disorders in Chinese society also problematize the connections between cultural institutions and universal psychiatric disorders. The emphasis on harmonious family and interpersonal relationships is identified as the main factor that influences mental health in Chinese society.[5] Arthur Kleinman's anthropological study of neurasthenia and depression in Chinese society is also typical. Traditional cultural values and norms are said to lead Chinese to suppress distressing emotions and somatize social and psychological problems, thus transforming a universal disease of depression into a culturally particular illness—neurasthenia.[6]

This "culture versus a universal disease" approach is problematic in several ways. First, local knowledge is measured against the Western conceptual categories understood as normative and universal; the difference is perceived as deviant from the norm and then explained by referring to local cultural beliefs and practices. Sometimes, the argument can go the other way around. A harmonious and therapeutic traditional culture is presented in contrast to disintegrated, alienating, and pathogenic modern society.[7] Either reflects the same orientalist imagination that constructs a cultural other "in terms of specifically Western discursive categories."[8] Second, as shown in recent medical anthropological studies, illness behavior and health-seeking strategies are complicated processes that respond to a complex of personal, social, and material exigencies and involve negotiating among diversified perspectives and resources available to patients and their families. To assume that people make rational decisions simply based on what they believe and explain the complexity of health and illness in terms of a few oversimplified cultural rules and beliefs offers an impoverished understanding of both culture and medicine.

My ethnographic account of emotion-related disorders in the context of Chinese medicine is informed by three different theoretical perspectives.

My approach to the Chinese experience of emotions and illness is inspired by the recent anthropological discourse of embodiment that locates culture in "the lived body" of everyday practice and directs analytical attention to the experiential aspect of culture in everyday life.[9] Culture is not simply understood in symbolic or structural terms as representations or abstract structures detached from bodily performance and presence.[10] Ethnographic writing has shown increased interest in "embodied culture." In her ethnography *Training the Body for China*, Brownell makes a compelling argument that "an ethnography account that overlooks the body omits the center of human experience."[11] Increasingly, medical anthropologists focus on "lived body" as a way to think and talk about illness and distress as they are experienced and to produce "experience-near" ethnographic accounts of suffering. Jenkins and Valient analyze the narratives of Salvadoran women to show *el calor* (heat) as a culturally specific body experience that is "existentially isomorphic with anger and fear."[12] Ots offers a semantic and phenomenological analysis of some of the most common symptoms presented in *zhongyi* clinics and explores the meanings of bodily perceptions both in *zhongyi* discourse and in patients' presentations. He suggests that the Chinese experience of body and emotion provides insight into the correspondence of emotions and bodily manifestations in emotion-affected disorders, and that bodily organs or emotional metaphors in Chinese medicine, such as "the angry liver," "the anxious heart," and "the melancholy spleen," "may serve as evidence for the role of the body in generating culture."[13]

Desjarlais, in an ethnography based on his field experience among the Yolmo of Nepal, proposes an analytical approach that attends to the "surface imagery, felt quality, and embodied values intrinsic to moments of illness and healing."[14] In my writing of *qingzhi* disorders, I pay similar attention to felt quality of culture that informs and gives styles and meaning to Chinese experience of pain and malaise. By attending to aesthetics of body-person (*shenti* 身体) that ordinary Chinese are tacitly oriented to in their everyday lives, my study explores the interplay among the bodily sensibilities, *zhongyi* constructions, and local social processes and gives a sense as to how it might "feel" for someone suffering a *qingzhi* disorder and the feeling of the heart-emotion (*xinqing* 心情) blocked from flowing and extending freely.

My research also draws extensively from current language theories that give primacy to language use in its social context. As Good and Good argue, any approach to studying illness and medicine, especially cross-culturally, has to address meaning and thus is embedded in a particular theory of language.[15] Ethnomedical research based on "emic" studies of folk nosologies[16] and combining "emic" categories with "etic" measures of biosciences[17] is grounded in the conventional theory of meaning[18] that links a word to an object or a concept. The medical discourse is therefore seen as establishing connections between a patient's pathological condition and a particular disease category. Accordingly, the meaning of a folk illness can be uncovered through a series of mappings, such as mapping "emic" symptom expressions onto the indigenous categories of illnesses, then onto the underlying physiological process, and finally onto the "etic" diagnostic entities of scientific medicine.[19] This referential approach to meaning and its application for cross-cultural comparisons have been faulted for its serious limitations in accounting for meanings in particular sociocultural contexts. As noted by many medical anthropologists, illness realities are never merely reflections of human biology but are socioculturally constituted and therefore need a different articulation of meaning.

Byron Good, in his study of "heart distress" in a small town in Iran, systematically records the domains of meaning associated with core symbols and symptoms in medical lexicon and reveals a configuration of meanings that associate old age, sorrow and sadness, ritual mourning, poverty, worries and anxiety, blood problems, and so on. He argues that "such a syndrome is not merely a reflection of symptoms linked with each other in natural reality, but a set of experiences associated through networks of meaning and social interaction in a society."[20] This conception of medical language directs research attention to the creative use of medical discourse in articulating experience of social distress and in negotiating meanings of suffering. Adding a critical dimension to this meaning-centered approach, some medical anthropologists argue that cultural analysis of illness and medicine have to take into consideration sociopolitical dimensions of power, interest, and resistance.[21] For these medical anthropologists, healing is also an ideological practice, and medicine can be analyzed as part of the social order, which also engages itself in the process of objectification and mystification of social facts, specifically, the process of medicalization of social problems and political oppression.[22] In her analysis of the disorder of nervosa among impoverished shantytown dwellers in northeast Brazil, Scheper-Hughes points to multiple meanings associated with the illness, such as a refusal of "demeaning and debilitating labor" and a response to violence and tragedy in everyday life.[23] Similarly, Kleinman & Kleinman analyze illness narratives of Chinese patients suffering chronic pains and emotional disorders to show the connection between physical complaints and political violence, personal or collective demoralization and delegitimization.[24]

My own research is aligned with the above outlined meaning-centered enterprise of medical anthropology but goes beyond the symbolic and semiotic dimensions of meaning by including interactive aspects of actual clinical encounters. If it is agreed that talking is an act that is socially effective, the interactive dimensions of social discourse—how a person presents and evaluates his/her own experience and how he/she is interpreted, understood, and responded to by others—offers a practical and useful way for understanding local experience in everyday life. Various medical discourse analyses, for example, demonstrate that a close examination of "talk" could be an effective tool to explore how illness realities are actually constructed and social roles and relations are enacted through clinical interactions.[25] Taking *zhongyi* clinical encounters as real-time sociolinguistic events, my ethnographic research incorporates microanalytical concepts and methods developed by various discourse analysis scholars[26] in examining interactive exchanges between doctors and patients during the routine clinical process of "looking at illness" (*kanbing* 看病) to trace and demonstrate how and at what point various clinical decisions were made and therapeutic transformations achieved. From this perspective, culture is examined as local processes and resources that members are oriented to from different subject positioning and that are evoked by the members in everyday social interactions to negotiate with and make sense of one another. It is in this mundane practice that culture is confirmed, contested, destabled, and transformed.

Finally, contemporary *zhongyi* scholar-physicians see their profession as built upon "a unique body of medical theories" (*dute de yixue lilun tixi* 独特的 医学理论体系) that is deeply rooted in "ancient [*gudai* 古代] Chinese people's scientific practice and philosophical thinking." In other words, Chinese medicine not only is grounded in collectively accumulated practical experience (*jinyan* 经验) but also owes as much to particular ways of thinking and theorizing. Classic Chinese philosophy and medical reasoning employ the same language, such as *yin-yang* and *wuxing* 五行 (five transformative phases) interactions and correlations as well as *qi* 气 (vital energy) transformations. This language evokes a world of transformation, in which myriad things and events are constantly in motion and extension and changes are seen as resulting from inherent complementary and contradictory *yin-yang* dynamics rather than resorting to any transcendental power or force essential in the Western intellectual traditions.[27] This particular way of philosophizing and theorizing is very much present in contemporary *zhongyi* texts and clinical reasoning under the name of rephrased "simple materialism and dialectic thinking" (*pusu weiwuzhuyi he bianzhengfa sixiang* 朴素唯物主义和辩证法思想). Any interpretation of Chinese medicine then has to be aware of the fundamental difference of the intellectual environment that has bred and nourished Chinese medicine and to be informed by classic Chinese cosmological assumptions distinctive from those underlying modern scientific thinking.[28]

It is this enriched meaning-centered interpretive approach combining analysis of local, interactive, and embodied meanings with a sensitivity to the epistemology and with a "civilization awareness"[29] that provides the general conceptual and methodological orientations of this book. It explores how indigenous Chinese medical concepts and knowledge related to *qingzhi* and its disorders are constructed, explained, and embodied in everyday *zhongyi* clinical practices and experiences. It also examines the interactive dimensions of medical and social discourse of *qingzhi* illnesses and analyzes how the *zhongyi* discourse links the illness construction to expressed and tacit cultural orientations, and how this indigenous illness category that recognizes simultaneously bodily, mental-emotional, and social experience in the illness provides meaningful forms of suffering for Chinese patients. Although I do not resort to reductive, objective, and standardized categories of comparison, I nevertheless see my study as comparative. For the ethnographic work to grasp the meaning of the "lived" life of a people and to convey it effectively to a reader who is linguistically and culturally alien to that people, the comparativeness must be already immanent in the ethnographic translation itself.

TOPIC ORIENTATIONS

Does Chinese medicine treat disordered emotions or emotional distresses? Contemporary *zhongyi* physicians seem unequivocal about Chinese medicine's role in treating disordered emotions. They insist that *zhongyi* has always paid considerable attention to emotional or psychosocial aspects in illness and health, and they could cite numerous examples from *zhongyi* classics to support this claim.[30] My own observations in Beijing confirmed that Chinese patients do habitually seek help in *zhongyi* clinics for what, in the West, might be considered psychological distress or a psychiatric disorder.[31] Typically, patients present their complaints in "bodily language,"[32] yet without denying affectivity as a source of their suffering. They take herbal remedies or other "traditional" forms of treatment[33] and claim to feel much better (*haoduo le* 好多了). Both patients and doctors of Chinese medicine with whom I interacted in Beijing insisted that *zhongyi* enjoys a special efficacy with such "functional disorders" (*gongneng xing jibing* 功能性疾病), while *xiyi* 西医 (literally, "Western medicine," referring to the biomedicine practiced in modern China) shows no effective means in treating such illnesses.

Yet, the question remains a problematic issue for anthropologists and scholars of Chinese medicine. For some, the topic is a slippery terrain that is better to be circumvented. The underlying concern is that Chinese medicine does not presuppose a dualistic separation of mind and body, nor does it typically make a categorical distinction between psychological and physical disorders,[34] therefore any discussion of *zhongyi* focusing on emotion inevitably makes modern clinical psychology or psychiatric medicine a comparative reference, thus imposing on Chinese medicine the structure of the Western biomedical model that typically views diseases as having a separate ontology as if they are either "in the body" or "in the mind."[35]

This is a legitimate concern. The ordinary Chinese terms for body, mind, and emotion do not evoke a simple divide between the physical and the psychological. *Shenti*, a word with a connotation of "person" and "self," is much more active and intentional than body, which etymologically is in English a physical "container" devoid of the mind.[36] *Shenti* is both physical and extraphysical, capable of feeling, perceiving, creating, and resonating or embodying changes and transformations in the social world as well as in the natural world. It is the world: at the same time, emotive, moral, aesthetic, and visceral. Neither is *jingshen* 精神[37] an equivalent to soul or spirit in English. It does not imply a disembodied mentality or a higher order of existence. In fact, *jingshen*, the combination of two characters of *jing* 精 (concentrated basis of vitality) and *shen* 神 (vitality as manifested through functional activities of mind and body), suggests a dynamic and inseparable relationship in the lived world of mind-body. Similarly, *xin* 心 is both heart and mind; *qingzhi* is also a process both mindful and visceral. These are not considered as essentially different kinds of existence[38] but different in functions or manifestations that are temporal and contingent.

In other words, the domains of body, mind, and emotion are mutually penetrating and activating. Such correlativity is embodied in the most mundane levels of everyday life, in the patterns and rhythms of work, exercising, eating, sleeping, and becoming ill and being healed. Apparently, Chinese medicine heals *qingzhi* disorders in a world that is not consistent with the epistemological structure of the Western biomedical model of knowing and practice.[39] Its practical logic involves a language of "bodies" in dynamic process and constant transformation and a language of relations. The *zhongyi* language of *yin-yang*, *jing* (concentrated basis for vitality), *qi* (vital energy), *shen* (vitality), *zangfu* 脏腑 (the visceral systems), *jingluo* 经络 (meridian tracts), has its roots in a distinctive cultural tradition and a unique history and evokes a different sense and experience of order and disorder. Its cultural and therapeutic efficacy evolves through a process of attuning (*tiao* 调), which in different clinical contexts is demonstrated as the actions of reordering (*li* 理), unblocking and freeing (*tong* 通), calming and neutralizing (*ping* 平), harmonizing and mediating (*he* 和) releasing and dissolving (*jie* 解), and so on.

Therefore, language itself becomes problematic and a subject of focus for this book. It seeks to understand *qingzhi* disorders as they are treated in the clinics of a *zhongyi* hospital on its own terms. In the words of my *zhongyi* teacher in Beijing, that means not to use a Western scientific way of thinking (*siwei fangshi* 思维方式) to frame *zhongyi* theory and practice but to understand how it really works within the relations between its own theory and practice (*zishen lilun he shijian de guanxi* 自身理论和实践的关系). The primary concern is not only to translate the relevant terms and concepts but also to make sense of a distinctive embodied experience of being ill and being healed.

For many scholars engaged in cross-culture psychiatric studies in Chinese society, *zhongyi*, because it does not recognize the separation of the mental from the physical, not only does not offer a legitimate way to treat an emotional distress but also exerts a negative cultural influence on developing a modern mental health care system for China.[40] Previous cross-cultural psychiatric and medical anthropological research on emotional distress and disorders was mostly carried out in the Western psychiatric context in Chinese society using biomedical models as the standard for comparative investigations.[41] Studies of this paradigm, in general, fail to assign any significant meaning to Chinese medicine in treating emotion-related disorders. They tend to interpret the way Chinese present, experience, and seek help for emotion-related disorders in terms of cultural beliefs and norms that emphasize somatic experience, "cognitive coping strategies" that patients and families employ to cope with highly stigmatized dysphoric affects, or simply cognitive and linguistic deficiency in expressing feelings.[42] In short, it is conceptualized as "somatization,"[43] a cultural process that transforms "an essential psychological event into a secondary somatic expression."[44]

Somatization has been seen as "a basic feature of the construction of illness in Chinese culture"[45] and for some time was alleged to be a "culture-specific trait typical of the Chinese people."[46] *Zhongyi* language is said to lack explicit terms for the description of emotional states and contributes to the somatization of affective illness among Chinese.[47] Tseng, too, argues that the characteristics of Chinese medicine, such as emphasis of visceral organs and the concepts of "exhaustion," "weakness," and "emptiness," strongly influence Chinese psychiatric patients.[48]

This book shares the cross-cultural psychiatric interest in emotion-related disorders in Chinese society; however, my research is of a different type. It is situated in a context of Chinese medicine, in which the basic psychiatric conception of "mental" versus "physical," "emotion" versus "cognitive," or "illness entity" versus "illness behavior" is questionable. I question applicability of the concept of somatization in Chinese experience. In fact, Chinese psychiatrists in actual clinical settings have no difficulty making connections between bodily and emotional changes as Chinese medical doctors habitually do. They agree that symptom expression, be it somatic or psychological, depends on how the individual experiences these changes at the specific moment and that Chinese patients do not limit their complaints to a somatic mode but present psychological and emotional symptoms too.[49] I also question the soundness of any national or community-based mental health policy and service in China that excludes zhongyi from playing an active role despite the fact that Chinese people routinely utilize zhongyi themselves in their fight against the illnesses allegedly emotional or mental according to the biomedical model.[50]

My study lies outside the paradigm of cross-culture psychiatry and asks different questions. Zhongyi doctors in the past and present do not have to resort to the underlying assumption of modern psychiatry—the dichotomy of mind and body—in order to understand and treat the disorders that predominantly involve emotions and thoughts. This does not mean that zhongyi clinicians have been unable to see the distinctions,[51] but rather their epistemological and professional "bias" emphasizes interconnections among emotions, thoughts, and various visceral systems. These underlying connections are actively explored by them as sources for fighting illnesses, physical as well as emotional. To zhongyi clinicians, disordered emotions or thoughts can have physiological consequences and vice versa, and a clinical intervention may start from either end or both. Then the questions are Does zhongyi's distinctive approach to disordered emotions and thoughts have any therapeutic value in contemporary China? If the answer is yes, how does it actually work clinically today? Can zhongyi be incorporated as effective resources into the national and community programs and services to improve mental health care for Chinese people? There is an applied dimension implied in this book. It shows that zhongyi has a unique role to play in its care for the emotionally ill and that social and mental health facilities can benefit from zhongyi's participation.

In my study, qingzhi disorder is seen as a zhongyi construct, complete and valid in itself, not a culturally mediated version of a "real" psychiatric disease. It is an ethnographic research without psychobiological measurements. Throughout the book, qingzhi disorder remains a Chinese experience: a meaningful form of suffering for those who seek to balance and to put back in order their upset world of shenti (body-person). Surely it is possible to compare qingzhi disorder with relevant psychiatric constructs of depression or anxiety, yet it requires a different type of research that goes beyond the frame and the scope of this book.

This book is not meant to offer a comprehensive account of the practice of Chinese medicine in contemporary China. Yet it is helpful to situate my own ethnographic investigation of qingzhi disorders in relation to some of the recent anthropological studies of Chinese medicine in contemporary China.

In the early 80s, Judith Farquhar spent eighteen months studying and conducting participant observation at the Guangzhou College of Traditional Chinese Medicine. Her book Knowing Practice: The Clinical Encounter of Chinese Medicine (1994) is based primarily on this experience. In the book, Farquhar discusses in great detail the process of "looking at illness" (*kanbing* 看病) in *zhongyi* clinical encounters and the practical logic of this process, which a *zhongyi* practitioner has to follow in order to effect healing. My study is indebted to her insights in clinical encounters of Chinese medicine, and I benefit from her discussions on the epistemological incompatibility between the biomedical sciences and Chinese medicine.

A number of factors set my study apart from hers. Farquhar makes extensive use of *zhongyi* textbooks and published cases for her analysis. My own study focuses mostly on the actual clinical work with all of its interactive implications. Second, the process of *kanbing* is understood as the process of doctor and patient looking at illness together. Farquhar's analysis is more directed to the professional point of view, that is, what a doctor needs to know in order to effect a cure. My study that takes a face-to-face interaction as a strategic site for understanding the clinical process presents both the professional and the patient's perceptions and shows the role that the patient plays in both the diagnosis and the healing. Finally, my focus is on *qingzhi* disorders where affective factors in Chinese medicine have received an ultimate attention, while in Farquhar's study, affectivity is not a topic of concern.

Any writing of Chinese medicine in contemporary China will inevitably confront the issue of plurality. Diversity is observable at every level of Chinese medical discourse and practice. The heterogeneity of Chinese medicine in the past and present has been widely described and commented on by scholars mostly in the West.[52] Chinese sources tend to take *zhongyi* pluralities for granted and see little need for further justification, whereas unity or uniformity is seen as something that needs to be established. Scholar-physicians of different schools in the past found their identity by tracing their professional genealogies to *Huangdi Neijing* 黄帝内经 (Yellow Emperor's Inner Classics), *Shanghan Lun* 伤寒论 (Discussions of Cold Damage), and other canonical texts, and to great masters in the history of Chinese medicine. For contemporary *zhongyi* scholars, there is not only a need to show continuity of their profession from the past but also a pressure to demonstrate its alignment with modern science. Interestingly, while the process of standardization (*guifanhua* 规范化) or systemization (*xitonghua* 系统化) based on biomedical models has significantly transformed the face of *zhongyi* organization and practice, original styles, personal experience, and individual virtuosity are continuously valued in the profession and deliberately sought by patients. In a sense, the participation of biomedicine adds more dimensions to the existing pluralities of Chinese medicine.[53]

Scholars of Chinese medicine in the West, from a different background in which existence of the objective truth is presupposed, are more likely to feel a compelling need to explain and justify diversity in Chinese medicine. In Elisabeth Hsu's ethnography, *The Transmission of Chinese Medicine*, the plurality is embedded in the transmission of knowledge in contemporary Chinese medicine. She shows that medical knowledge acquired through different modes of transmission and within different social relationships is understood and "known" differently. She describes three different modes of knowledge transmission in correspondence with three distinctive social settings, namely, the transmission of "secret knowledge" within a master-disciple relationship, "the personal transmission of knowledge" between a mentor and a follower characteristic of classical scholarship, and "the standardized mode of transmission" in the context of modern classroom learning.[54] Volker Scheid takes plurality and diversity as the main thesis of his book, *Chinese Medicine in Contemporary China: Plurality and Synthesis*, which examines "a plurality of agencies and processes involved in the shaping of contemporary Chinese medicine," including politicians and state, patients and physicians, classical scholarship and modern health care systems, institutions, networks, and training of *zhongyi* physicians.[55] In my own ethnography, plurality is not a topic but a context. I take Scheid's conclusion that plurality is "an intrinsic aspect of contemporary Chinese medicine"[56] as a starting point and explore how multiple perspectives and sources of knowledge play out in an actual clinical process. In this sense, my case studies of *qingzhi* disorders should be read as an analysis of a microprocess of a local synthesis rather than as an attempt to provide a complete or comprehensive presentation of how *qingzhi* disorders are diagnosed and treated generally in clinics of Chinese medicine.

ETHNOGRAPHIC SETTINGS

After being away from China for about four years, I went back to Beijing in January 1994 to conduct a twelve-month fieldstudy for my ethnographic study on emotion-related disorders in the clinics of Chinese medicine, on which this book is based. However, my research for the book has continued beyond the original fieldwork through correspondence and interactions with *zhongyi* professionals and scholars both in and outside China, as well as subsequent visits to the original field sites and through reading the published literature on Chinese medicine.

For this anthropological research, I relied heavily on participant observation as well as semistructured and unstructured interviews with patients, doctors, and ordinary Chinese citizens, whom I came to know by different means and at different times. My own personal background as a Chinese native who grew up and was educated in China permitted me ready access to the Chinese cultural resources and social networks, which were very much needed in doing such research. Needless to say, however, the way I formulated my theoretical positions and interpreted the empirical data and the way in which I actually went about doing my interviews and observations bore the cultural and experiential marks of me as a Western trained native anthropologist.

My fieldwork took me to various hospitals and clinics of Chinese medicine in Beijing, but the major part of the clinical observation was carried out in one of the affiliated hospitals of the Beijing Academy of Chinese Medicine. The hospital was built in the mid-1950s. Over the decades, it has been expanded and developed into one of the largest *zhongyi* hospitals as well as a major clinical research and teaching center for Chinese medicine in the Beijing area. Many physicians who work in the hospital divide their time among clinical work, research, and teaching. Clearly my ethnographic account of clinical encounters reflects the practice of this elite and professionalized Chinese medicine, which, as an integrated part of the national health care system, is sanctioned and closely supervised by the state.

The organization and management of the hospital resembles, in every important way, a modern biomedical hospital in Beijing. It consists of 24 clinical departments (*ke-shi* 科室), including *qigong* 气功 (breathing exercises for improving health or curing disease) and *zhenjiu* 针灸 (acupuncture and moxibustion) clinics that are not common divisions in most biomedical hospitals in China, and 13 labs and research departments of medical sciences and technology, which centrally reflect the policy of "using modern science and technology to conduct scientific research of traditional Chinese medicine."[57] I chose Shenjing Ke 神经科 (Clinic of Neuropathic Disorders) as the primary site for my clinical observations.[58] Like many other structural categories in a modern *zhongyi* hospital, the name of Shenjing Ke itself came from the biomedical model in an attempt to establish greater authority in the culture of modern science. The reason I chose Shenjing Ke as the base of my research is mainly because it has a large concentration of patients with *qingzhi* disorders. When referring to an illness, ordinary Chinese do not typically make distinctions between "of nerves" (*shenjing* 神经) and "of mind or spirit" (*jingshen* 精神). Chinese use "neurological disorder" (*shenjing bing* 神经病) casually to mean "mental illness" (*jingshen bing* 精神病). The doctors I worked with in this particular clinic estimated that about 75 % of their patients who came to seek medical help suffered a *qingzhi* related disorder. In addition, the director of the clinic is recognized as an expert in treating such disorders, especially, stagnation syndrome (*yuzheng* 郁证), in which I was particularly interested.

I was introduced to the head of the clinic, who is a senor doctor known for his efficacy in treating *qingzhi* disorders, through a mutual friend. At our first meeting, he emphasized that *zhongyi* and *xiyi* (Western biomedicine) are of two different "ways of thinking" (*siwei fangshi* 思维方式) and that I should be cautious not to interpret *zhongyi* simply in terms of Western scientific categories and language. According to him, a good understanding of *zhongyi* requires a completely different language, and it takes time to slowly "understand through direct experience" (*tihui* 体会) *zhongyi* theories and practices. I could not agree more with this advice. A good rapport between the senior doctor and me started from this straightforward conversation. I was later given permission to do participant observations in his clinic. In an anthropological expression, I was "adopted" into the community by assuming a student role. The doctor took it to be his responsibility to see that I really understood Chinese medical concepts and clinical actions so that I would not misrepresent Chinese medicine in my research. I followed the doctor in his clinic for about ten months like one of his student doctors, though I did not wear their uniform. As a result, I became familiar with his colleagues working in the same consulting room, his graduate students, and some of his patients. Most of all, I gained considerable *tihui* of Chinese medicine. Toward the end of my fieldwork, my doctor friends told me that I used their language and asked "correct" questions, and they joked that I could even open a clinic of Chinese medicine myself some day.

During my clinical observations, I recorded more than four hundred cases. The procedure was to sit beside the doctor, take notes, and later with the participants' permission to record clinical interactions. I was encouraged to move along with the clinical process, when appropriate, to feel a patient's pulse, look at his/her tongue, and ask questions. Sometimes, the doctor would directly put me on the spot by suggesting that a patient talk with me, and he introduced me as an anthropologist doing a research project on emotion-related disorders. Only a few patients actually agreed to sit down for an interview. Most patients would simply decline the invitation citing various reasons. Most of my interviews of patients were semistructured and took place outside the clinical room. The questions centered on the informants' illness history and experience as well as their *zhongyi* knowledge. The purpose of my questions was to understand a patient perspective on his or her illness and the role of emotion in his or her illness experience and also to record patients' narratives regarding how they coped with and accounted for or made sense of their sufferings, and why they chose to see a *zhongyi* doctor. My one disappointment was that I was not able to build up a closer rapport and have more in-depth interviews with the patients. Conducting an interview with a patient proved to be challenging and, sometimes, frustrating. Partly this was due to the clinical settings of my research. Patients came to the clinic for treatment because they were suffering. They had little time or interest in talking to a stranger, much less talking about their personal lives beyond their immediate concerns of their illnesses. I also felt little justified to probe into a patient's personal life. In fact, *zhongyi* doctors are very subtle when coming to sensitive personal questions. I was told that a doctor should not probe into anything that a patient was deliberately avoiding talking about, because that could only add stress and anxiety to the patient and interfere with the efficacy of the therapy. This is especially a concern with patients who suffer from a *qingzhi* disorder. However, I was able to carry out lengthy and in-depth interviews with the patients whom I happened to know well and friends and relatives who suffered emotion-related disorders and sought Chinese medical treatment.

My experience with doctors was quite different. I saw them several times a week and had lunch with them at the hospital's cafeteria. They were interested in my experiences in the United States. My interaction with them was informal and relaxed. Unstructured interviews were carried out with them whenever it was convenient. These interviews covered broad medical, social, cultural, and political topics, as well as personal experiences.[59]

My participant observation also went beyond the major field site. Directly under the Ministry of Health, this hospital closely reflects the official policies to promote *zhongyi* to a modern scientific realm and to explore ways to combine Western and Chinese medicines. In terms of funding and other forms of government support, it has advantages over many other smaller hospitals. My experience in other Chinese medical institutions that are less prestigious provided a comparative perspective.

Coming back to the much changed neighborhood in the Haidian district where I used to live, I was impressed by the number of *zhongyi* clinics in the neighborhood. Within the area where I live, there were two *zhongyi* outpatient clinics with a Chinese pharmacy attached, a small *zhongyi* hospital, a *zhongyi* clinic within a community hospital, and a new *zhongyi* consulting room added to a health clinic. I frequented these smaller Chinese medical institutions, especially the small *zhongyi* hospital, which lay hidden in a small lane behind tall buildings. The hospital specialized in treating chronic and difficult diseases (*manxing yinan bingzheng* 慢性疑难病证) by combining Chinese and Western medicines (*zhong-xi yi jiehe* 中西医结合). I was surprised to find a *Jingshen Ke* 精神科 (mental health clinic) in this small hospital, which was not a common division in *zhongyi* hospitals. From the information provided in the various posters, pictures, and banners in this location, I recognized quite a few names of famous senior doctors (*laozhongyi* 老中医) and professors, who were invited to work part time there, while keeping their permanent positions in other hospitals and research or teaching institutes. Their presence made this small hospital popular. Some of my interviews with patients were carried out in this small hospital.

The economic reforms that gained momentum in the 1980s and the movement toward the free market system have changed the face of *zhongyi* practice in an important way. The new economic policies have encouraged the flow of *zhongyi* knowledge and practitioners from the large state institutions to smaller community clinics and private hospitals.[60] Not only do well-established senior doctors run their own private clinics, but the young graduates of *zhongyi* colleges and universities may also engage in sideline businesses.[61] Between large state-sponsored institutions and smaller or privately owned practices, there is no strict boundary but a constant flow of knowledge and resources.

During my residency in Beijing, I stayed in a community where my parents lived and where families had known one another for a long time and shared many social occasions. In this community I was a true participant in every sense, visiting my neighbors, helping out and being helped, listening to gossip in the mail room, and talking to people while taking a walk in the neighborhood parks. Not only did I observe daily social and emotional interactions and actual management of emotional crisis and illnesses, but I was also sometimes part of that process. Former classmates, friends, and relatives were also valuable resources for my research. I was given access to their medical records and prescriptions and was allowed to accompany them to see a doctor. With them, I carried out lengthy and in-depth interviews regarding their personal and emotional experience. I understood them and shared many of their worries, anxieties, confusions, and hopes.

THE FRAMEWORK OF THE BOOK

In this introduction, I have outlined some theoretical and conceptual considerations that are central to a cultural understanding of *qingzhi* disorders in contemporary practice of Chinese medicine and introduced the ethnographic subjects and settings. I situate my research in the anthropological discourse of body, emotion, illness, and medicine. I show how my study is related to and different from other relevant studies theoretically and empirically. Chapter 2 discusses the continuity and modern transformation of Chinese medicine. One purpose of this chapter is to historicize the form of *zhongyi* practice in contemporary China. It explores how the manifold historical events and forces since the late nineteenth century have been at work in shaping the traditional indigenous "*yi* (medicine)" into present day cosmopolitan *zhongyi*. This chapter also seeks to ground "modern" *zhongyi* in an epistemological tradition that approaches knowledge, theory, and practice differently from that of the modern Western science and that gives Chinese medicine a sense of continuity from its distant and recent past. Chapter 3 explores the Chinese world of body-person (*shenti*), through the analysis of cultural semantics and aesthetics of *shenti* embodied in the way Chinese talk about their body and experience the "loss of balance" (*shitiao* 失调) or "being in discord" (*weihe* 违和). I show that the way Chinese patients experience *qingzhi* disorders and the Chinese medical therapeutic process in healing them are profoundly embedded in the cultural sensibilities and the meanings of body, person, and society. In other words, the cultural aesthetics and values persistent in Chinese society are embodied and are thus particularly visible when the body-person is in "dis-ease." Chapter 4, focusing specifically on the Chinese concept of "*qingzhi*" (emotion-mind), explores the sociocultural and ethnomedical contexts where *qingzhi* and disordered *qingzhi* are formulated, talked about, and experienced. Chapters 5 and 6 examine the meaning and the categorization of *qingzhi* disorders in relation to the *zhongyi* clinical process of "differentiation of syndromes and determination of therapies" (*bianzheng lunzhi* 辩正论治). Chapter 7 offers a close examination of an actual face-to-face clinical interaction, which shows how the syndrome of a particular *qingzhi* disorder is defined through ordinary clinical work and how the process of *tiao* (attuning) works to transform the patient's experience. Finally, Chapter 7 offers some general conclusions based on previous analysis and discussions. It is evident that *qingzhi* disorders—illnesses resulted from disordered emotions and social difficulties—in contemporary Chinese medicine offer a meaningful form and a viable language for Chinese patients to make sense of their sufferings and a practicable regimen to manage a lived body that falls out of order.

Throughout the book, Chinese medicine is used interchangeably with *zhongyi* to refer to the professional Chinese medicine practiced in contemporary China and its classic form of scholarly medicine, from which the present day *zhongyi* has evolved and transformed. Accordingly, *xiyi* and Western medicine, its direct translation, are also used interchangeably to refer to the form of biomedicine practiced in modern China. Translation of Chinese medical terminology proves to be a difficult task. My translation does not follow one single source. Instead, I consulted various sources[62] and decided on the ones I feel best reflect my understanding of the terms in the context. In other words, the translation itself may not be mine, but the choice is. Some Chinese terms are used untranslated, such as *qi* and *yin-yang*, which have been largely accepted as English words. For other commonly used terms that appear repeatedly in this book and of which no simple English translation is sufficient to capture an array of meanings, such as *qingzhi*, I tend to use the original Chinese term in *pinyin* transcript, which is supplemented with a suggested English translation at least when it appears for the first time in the chapter. Chinese characters of the term are also provided at least once in a chapter. I appreciate the challenge that this makes for non-Chinese readers, but I feel that it was important to include Chinese characters for those readers who read Chinese and depend on characters for specific meanings and sources of the terms.

Chinese Medicine:
Continuity and Modern Transformations

Although I did not expect to find "pure" Chinese medicine in practical clinical work, observing doctors in *zhongyi* 中医 (Chinese medicine) clinics handling the results of various biomedical tests and examinations with considerable confidence and skill was impressive. *Zhongyi* doctors and students I met in Beijing tend to see *zhongyi* and *xiyi* 西医 (Western medicine) as complementary and that both have their particular strengths (*youshi* 优势) in treating illnesses. They agree that nowadays, a good *zhongyi* doctor has to be knowledgeable in *xiyi* as well. Patients also seem to lack respect for the boundaries between these two different medical practices. They do not hesitate to show *zhongyi* doctors the results of their recent electroencephalograms or CAT scans and to discuss their previous clinical encounters in biomedical hospitals. *Zhongyi* physicians are expected not only to understand biomedical test results but also to be able to use biomedical concepts and terms.[1] They, too, sometimes order laboratory tests for a patient and take his/her blood pressure or prescribe biomedicines, often at a patient's request.[2] The influence of modern science and its epistemology on the practice and organization of professional Chinese medicine has been so extensive that the very identity of *zhongyi* practice as "traditional medicine" (*chuantong yixue* 传统医学) calls for reflection.

Moreover, Chinese people do not seem to be confused at all as to which system is Chinese and which is not. *Zhongyi* versus *xiyi* remains a significant distinction recognized by both medical professionals and the general population. Patients choose to utilize *zhongyi* or *xiyi*, or a combination of both[3] according to commonly recognized features of the different medical systems in relation to their specific illnesses or illness episodes, knowledge, previous experiences, and other practical concerns, such as cost and convenience. Judith Farquhar, in her book *Knowing Practice*, argues for "historical toughness" and epistemological distinctiveness of this non-Western healing practice.[4] "The practical logic" of *zhongyi* and "its ways of seeking efficacy" observed by Farquhar in the 1980s remained largely true in the 1990s when my study began. The present situation of *zhongyi* has to be understood both in its continuity as a body of medical knowledge and practices that have been evolving for more than two thousand years and as the product of the particular historical moment of the modern era.

MODERN TRANSFORMATIONS

Before Western medicine began to stream into China in the latter half of the nineteenth century, the indigenous medicine in China was simply called "*yi*" (medicine). Historically, *yi* coexisted and interacted with other healing practices, such as shamanic and religious healings. The boundaries among them in practice might not be clear cut. However, it was documented that as early as the Spring and Autumn of the Zhou Dynasty (770–476 BCE) *yi* had acquired an identity distinctive from *wu* 巫 or *zhu* 祝 (shamanic/spiritual healing) in its therapeutic rationalization and technology.[5] *Yi* 医 (medicine), as the historical source of today's *zhongyi*, refers mainly to a body of accumulated healing knowledge and practices based on a naturalistic explanation of disease and health rationalized in the language of "yin-yang" 阴阳 and "*wuxing*" 五行 (the five transformative phases),"[6] and "passed down by China's educated elite."[7]

The 1949 founding of the People's Republic of China is commonly recognized as the significant historical moment that marked a drastic transition in *zhongyi* practice and education in China. According to the contemporary Chinese historical narratives, before the Liberation (founding of PRC in 1949), *zhongyi* was "on the verge of dying out" (*binlin miewang* 濒临灭亡) under the old national government's discriminating policies against *zhongyi*, and it was with the establishment of the New China that *zhongyi* "acquired a new life" (*huode xinsheng* 获得新生).[8] In the past, most traditional Chinese medical doctors were individual practitioners working in their private clinics and pharmacies (often not completely separated from their living quarters). The practice was generally inherited within a family or passed down from a master to disciples. The beginning of the twentieth century witnessed increasing *zhongyi* activities in establishing academies and hospitals, organizing professional groups, and standardizing the knowledge. However, lacking in governmental support and endorsement, these activities remained largely weak and localized.

The modern institutionalization of Chinese medicine started in the mid-1950s. The Chinese Academy of Traditional Chinese Medicine, the first *zhongyi* institution directly under the Ministry of Public Health, was set up on December 19, 1955, through the merging of five different medical and research institutions. The hospital where I did most of my field research was one of the two *zhongyi* hospitals affiliated with the academy. They were among the first few *zhongyi* hospitals and colleges established in the mid-1950s. In 1956, four *zhongyi* colleges were established respectively in Beijing, Shanghai, Guangzhou, and

Chengdu to train advanced Chinese medical doctors and pharmacists. Following this trend, many provincial governments established their own higher educational institutions of Chinese medicine. At the same time, the individual practitioners of Chinese medicine who had been working in private clinics were invited to treat patients in hospitals, and many of them were assimilated into the different levels of public health institutions. "The diverse and scattered practitioners of traditional medicine, with their small academies and family clinics, were organized into a rapidly growing national hierarchy of clinical and academic institutions."[9]

However, to understand the contemporary situation of *zhongyi* in China, we should also pay attention to the manifold historical forces that have been at work in shaping *yi* into today's *zhongyi* since the second half of the nineteenth century when China was transformed abruptly into a shattered semicolonial society.

The practice of Western medicine in China before the second half of the nineteenth century was practically insignificant.[10] It did not pose a serious challenge to Chinese medicine until the turn of the century when Western medicine, armed with modern experimental science and imported into China together following the Western military powers and the Christian God,[11] established its permanent presence in China. However, for many reform-minded intellectuals and revolutionaries, what Western medicine offered at the turn of the century was not as much effective healing as the promise of Western scientific culture for national salvation.[12] The decades of humiliation following the brutal encounter with the modern Western civilization set many intellectuals to search for "salvation" beyond the boundary of their own civilization. Western science became a powerful intellectual resource that the Chinese reformists and revolutionaries drew on for an extensive cultural criticism of their own tradition, reaching its climax in the May 4 movement in 1919. "Mr. Science" (Sai Xiansheng 赛先生), as well as "Mr. Democracy" (De Xiansheng 德先生), became an overwhelming voice in twentieth-century China, so powerful that, as Hu Shi declared in 1923, "there is not a single person who calls himself a modern man and yet dares openly to belittle science."[13]

Within this historical atmosphere, the tension and polarity between Chinese and Western learning were obvious. This can be seen in the labels that identified traditional Chinese scholarship as "Chinese learning" (*zhongxue* 中学), "national learning" (*guoxue* 国学), or "old learning" (*jiuxue* 旧学), the Western knowledge as "Western learning" (*xixue* 西学) or "new learning" (*xinxue* 新学). Accordingly, indigenous medicine (*yi*) became "Chinese medicine" (*zhongyi* 中医), "national medicine" (*guoyi* 国医), or "old medicine" (*jiuyi* 旧医), while the biomedicine became "Western medicine" (*xiyi* 西医) or "new medicine" (*xinyi* 新医).[14] Building a strong "new China" under the guidance of a scientific spirit has been the dominant national sentiment from the beginning of the twentieth century to the present. It is reiterated in the contemporary discourse of the Four Modernizations, which draws heavily from the historical experience of the Chinese people at the turn of the century. The phrase backwardness incurring humiliation (*luohou jiuyao aida* 落后就要挨打) is a frequently used rhetoric in both official and popular discourse.

During the Republic period, attempts at eliminating *zhongyi* were a constant threat to the *zhongyi* profession. *Zhongyi*, seen as a partner of the old feudal culture and incompatible with modern scientific thinking, was an obstacle on the way to "wholehearted-modernization." In 1914 Wang Daxie, the minister of education of the government of Northern warlords (1912–27), declared that "[the government] had made up its mind to eliminate the traditional Chinese medical system and discard the use of Chinese material medica."[15] On the occasion of the first convention of the Central Committee for Public Health of the Kuomingtang government in 1929, a few members of a committee headed by Yu Yunxiu presented a motion to "wipe out obstacles in hygiene work by eliminating the traditional Chinese medicine system."[16] Many intellectuals within the Communist Party in the 1920s and 30s also argued vigorously against traditional medicine.[17]

In the decades of adversity, *zhongyi*, in resistance to official and elite pressure and in adaptation to the competition of *xiyi* for economic and political resources, transformed itself in several important ways. First, when facing the external challenge of an alien knowledge system of Western medicine, the internal tension among diverse doctrines and interpretations of Chinese medicine was reduced. Prior to its encounter with Western medicine, Chinese medicine from the Song-Yuan period (960–1368 AD) was characterized by tension between different schools of medical doctrines.[18] Especially, from the end of the Ming dynasty (1368–1644 AD) when the school of febrile/warm illnesses (*wenbing xuepai* 温病学派) emerged, the competition and even hostility between the school of cold damage illnesses (*shanghan* 伤寒) and the febrile/warm illness (*wenbing* 温病) school became increasingly furious as if they were as "incompatible as water and fire."[19] The reduction of internal tension was due as much to intentional efforts to form a united front against encroachment of Western medicine as to the fact that in reference to Western medicine, the common intellectual foundations and shared qualities of the different schools of Chinese medicine suddenly stood out. The differences in knowledge inheritance, in interpretation of medical concepts in the classics, and in emphasis on particular illness factors (*bingyin* 病因) and illness mechanisms (*bingji* 病机) became less significant. Focusing on the common characters of Chinese medicine in antithesis to Western medicine, the knowledge of Chinese medicine was inevitably reconstructed and shaped into a more coherently represented body of knowledge. The rhetoric of "contention between different schools of medical thought" (*xuepaizhizheng* 学派之争) was overshadowed by the discourse of *zhongyi* versus *xiyi*.

Second, in reaction to the official attempts to delegitimize the practice and teaching of *zhongyi* in the 1920s and 30s, the *zhongyi* practitioners and pharmacists were mobilized to stage national protests, which did force the government to step back from its radical policies to abandon Chinese medicine.[20] These protests also led to the establishment of the national organization of Chinese medicine.[21] *Zhongyi* at this moment began to see emergent professional communities and institutions. In the two decades between the 1920s and 30s, about seventy *zhongyi* schools and ninety *zhongyi* professional organizations were set up nationally. Although these institutions were still largely regional, their influences cut across the boundaries maintained in the past by the vertical relationship between masters and disciples, and the practitioners became aware of their common identity as *zhongyi* (Chinese medical practitioners).[22]

Finally, many analyses of Chinese medicine of this period emphasize the theme of nationalism, which identified *zhongyi* as "national essence" (*guocui* 国粹) and thus an important basis for its modern legitimacy.[23] In the case of *zhonyi*, however, the voice of preserving "national essence" did not go far. It was ridiculed as conservative and unpractical both before and after 1949. After all, the success of *zhongyi* could not be based solely on its "antiqueness" that needed to be preserved, but lay in its value as a practiced and organized way against diseases comparable to Western medicine in the modern world. The voices that had lasting influence on the modern form of *zhongyi* came from the discussions and publications that focused on integrating *zhongyi* and *xiyi* (*zhongxiyi huitong* 中西医汇通) represented by renowned Chinese physicians, such as Zhang Xichun (1860–1933) and Yun Tieqiao (1878–1935). Yun realized that "*zhongyi* has no way out but to deal with Western medicine" and that "*zhongyi* has demonstrated its capacity of integrating and evolving, and it will surely absorb the strength of *xiyi*, and integrate it into its system to form a new *zhongyi*."[24] Although how to integrate Chinese and Western medicines remained a debate for a long time to come, erudite Chinese physicians recognized the need for change. They expected to see a "new Chinese medicine" emerge from communication and convergence with the strengths of Western medicine. This articulation of the combination of Chinese medicine and Western medicine continues to inform the discourse and practice of Chinese medicine today.

As discussed above, the full legitimization and institutionalization of Chinese medicine in the early 1950s and the later years under the government's supporting policies was not without historical basis. However, compared to indigenous medical practices in other Asian societies and in other parts of the world, the ideological support for *zhongyi* education and practice from the new government by the Communist Party was unprecedented. In fact, the first generation of leadership of PRC, including Mao Zedong, Zhou Enlai, and Liu Shaoqi, gave instructions regarding incorporating *zhongyi* into the formal health care systems of the new society.[25] At the First National Conference on Health held in 1950, Mao called for "uniting all the health care workers, the old and new, Chinese and Western, to form a strong united front line for the cause of people's health." The principle of "uniting Chinese and Western medical professionals" (*tuanjie zhongxiyi* 团结中西医), and later "giving equal emphasis to both Chinese and Western medicines" (*zhongxiyi bingzhong* 中西医并重)

has been the basic approach to developing the dual state health system. Mao's famous comment of 1958 that "Chinese medicine and pharmaceutics are a great treasure house, and (we) must make all efforts to uncover it and raise its standard"[26] has been frequently quoted to give *zhongyi* an official voice and political status.

Chinese writings on modern *zhongyi* history tend to credit the Chinese Communist Party (CCP)'s "historical materialistic attitude toward the cultural legacy" (*dui wenhua yichan de lishi weiwuzhuyi taidu* 对文化遗产的历史唯物主义态度) with much of the responsibility for the fast growing of *zhongyi* after the establishment of the PRC. It is said that such a historicism recognizes the value of *zhongyi* as accumulated knowledge and experience against diseases throughout a long history of "practices of the masses" and calls for "inheriting" (*jicheng* 继承) and "developing or carrying forward" (*fazhan* 发展) the traditional Chinese medicine.

The new government's strong support for *zhongyi* also came from practical considerations. At the time when the Communists took power, the country's public health situation was appalling, and biomedical resources were scarce and unevenly distributed.[27] Scholars are generally convinced that the formidable task for the new government to provide a large population with basic health care motivated the policy makers to bring the traditional Chinese medical practitioners into the public health construction. One of the most effective approaches that characterized the revolution led by the CCP was the emphasis on mobilizing the masses, that is, working with whatever forces possible to form "a united front" (*tongyi zhanxian* 统一战线) against the main enemy of the time. At the time, Chinese medicine, which did not have the elite status of Western medicine, was more aligned with the masses to be mobilized and incorporated into the public health programs. The slogan of *tuanjie zhongyi* 团结中医 (uniting with Chinese medical workers) thus was not just a pragmatic strategy but also a politically significant move. Moreover, combining Western and Chinese medicines for a practical health care purpose was nothing new for the CCP.[28] The Communist Party, in its long period of armed resistance, accumulated experience of having both Chinese and Western doctors work together in its base areas. The policy to encourage both Chinese and Western doctors to learn from each other (*huxiang xuexi* 互相学习) worked well to produce a cooperative relationship between the Chinese and Western doctors, which was not found outside CCP's liberated bases (*jiefangqu* 解放区).[29] Arguably, the combination of Western and Chinese medicines (*zhong-xiyi jiehe* 中西医结合) for practical purpose has been largely a continuous health care policy for the CCP, although it has not gone without controversies at the theoretical level.[30]

As shown above, the drastic transformation of Chinese medicine after 1949—the hospital-based practice, standardization of knowledge, and classroom-centered education,—was built upon continuous changes that happened during the Republic era or even earlier. The move to modernize and scientize Chinese medicine had started long before the 1950s.[31] *Zhongyi* professionals, particularly those well-known physicians and staunch advocates of *zhongyi* practice and education in the 1920s and 30s, were willing participants and active agencies in the process of *zhongyi* transformation in the 1950s. As Scheid notes, many of them "became key players in the shaping of Chinese medicine after 1954."[32] In addition, the newly acquired political status and professional space in the official health care system further motivated the *zhongyi* community to align with the political and practical goals of the new government.

THE PROBLEM OF THEORY
AND CONTINUITY OF CHINESE MEDICINE

Modern *zhongyi* writings habitually make discursive connections between the present practices and past achievements to highlight the continuity of the present from the ancient. Discussions of *zhongyi* basic theories inevitably cite the *Huangdi Neijing* 黄帝内经 (Yellow Emperor's Inner Classics)[33] for laying out the theoretical foundations of Chinese medicine.[34] Similarly, the exposition of formulas (*fangjixue* 方剂学) consistently credits the ancient books on formulas (*jingfang* 经方), especially Zhang Zhongjing's *Shanghan Zabing Lun* 伤寒雜 病论 (Discussions of Cold Damage and various Disorders) for setting up the basics for Chinese medical formulas.[35]

For many Western scholars of Chinese medicine, the stories told by the Chinese physicians at best constitute an imagined continuity or a false impression that the so-called *zhongyi* consists of a well-defined, unified, and coherent system of knowledge comparable to the Western biomedicine and "basically unchanged since antiquity."[36] To them, this tradition has been marked by conceptual contradictions, heterogeneous origins, historical ruptures, and continuous adjustments to sociopolitical changes.[37] Any historical narrative is a form of construction; the story of the evolution of Chinese medicine is not an exception. However, to assume *zhongyi* scholars' emphasis on continuity and connections inevitably entails a denial of diversity and changes is a misreading reflecting the Western epistemological bias that dichotomizes unity (*tongyi* 同 一) and diversity (*chayi* 差异).

From the perspective of the Chinese correlative way of thinking evident in the Chinese philosophic reflections and historical discourses, continuity and creativity or unity and diversity presuppose each other. They are viewed as interdependent, thus forming a pair of complementary oppositions. For instance, *Shanghai Lun* (Discussion of Cold Damage) is considered another paramount achievement in the history of Chinese medicine after the publication of *Neijing* (the Inner Classics). Its author, Zhang Zhongjing, an East Han physician, was said to have produced the highly innovative treatise on treating cold-damage related and other disorders, drawing on his intensive studies of various medical texts of and before his time, including the classic *Neijing*. His accomplishment is often talked about in terms of continuity from the previous monumental achievements, such as *Neijing*. Yet the content of

Shanghan Lun shows an obviously different approach from *Neijing*. *Neijing*'s discussions of "meridian channels" (*jingluo* 经络) and "visceral organ systems" (*zangfu* 脏腑) feature little in Zhongjing's "six patterns of diagnosis" (*liujing bianzheng* 六经辨证). The theoretical elaboration of *wuxing* 五行 (five transformative phases) found in *Neijing* is completely absent from *Shanghan Lun*.[38] However, he drew freely from the ancient texts on formulas (*jingfang*). By virtue of the differences, innovations, and physician's unique synthesis of the past knowledge with his own clinical practices and experiences, *Shanghan Lun* positions itself in a particular relationship to *Neijing* and therefore constitutes a continuity that not only brings the past to the present but also opens new directions for the future. This correlative way of explaining the transformative process of Chinese medicine can be found in the classic Chinese thought of "continuity through changes" (*tongbian* 通变) traceable to the earliest Chinese philosophic reflections in *Yijing* 易经 (Book of changes)[39] and in the language of "inheriting" (*jicheng* 继承) and "developing/carrying forward" (*fazhan* 发展) of the modern discourse of "historical materialism" (*lishi weiwuzhuyi* 历史唯物主义).

Interestingly, the different explanation and use of medical concepts and the innovative clinical approaches in *Shanghan Lun* are not viewed by Chinese scholar-physicians as something invalidating the *Neijing* teachings; similarly, the *Neijing* doctrines are not used as the basis to judge and disqualify *Shanghan Lun*. Both are equally esteemed for offering valid and invaluable theoretical and practical guidance for *zhongyi* clinical work and have been studied diligently by generations of Chinese scholar-physicians. In fact, Chinese medical classics are marked by a lack of consistency and, sometimes, by obvious disagreements.[40] Yet Chinese physicians seem to take the diversity for granted and are not concerned much by seemingly conflicting statements in the medical theories. Such is the case. The articulation of theory (*lilun* 理论) within Chinese medicine therefore merits critical attention.

Modern *zhongyi* scholar-physicians never fail to stress that *zhongyi* possesses "a distinctive body of theories" (*dute de lilun tixi* 独特的理论体系) grounded in 2000 years of practice (*shijian* 实践), embodied in ever-increasing canonical texts (*jingdian lunzhu* 经典论著), and manifested in the virtuosity of exemplary physicians (*dayi* 大医). Experienced senior physicians of the modern time invariably emphasize the relevance of Chinese medical theories (*lilun* 理论) in clinical practices.[41] Senior doctors sometimes complain that the younger generation of Chinese medical doctors has not paid sufficient attention to *zhongyi* theories. My *zhongyi* teacher claimed that the questions and even the sequence of questions he asks during a clinical consultation are not random at all; like the therapeutic actions he chooses and the formulas he designs, all have a theoretical basis (*lilun genju* 理论根据). He frequently cautioned his student doctors who were busy taking notes that it would not help with their clinical work no matter how many formulas they took down if they did not understand the underlying logic of his questions and his therapeutic decisions. The senior doctor's claim was sometimes verified by younger doctors' frustrations. My friend, Dr. Wang, once complained, "We use a senior doctor's formula the same way as he did, but we never get the same effect." Then, what do Chinese scholar-physicians actually mean when they talk about *zhongyi lilun* (Chinese medical theories) or simply *yili* 医理 (medical theories), and in what sense these *lilun* are considered "distinctive."

The Chinese character *li* 理 has the meaning of naturally formed patterns or relations within the dynamic process of things (*shiwu* 事物). As a verb, *li* means to "trace out" or "map out" the "correlated details and the extended pattern of relationships."[42] *Lilun* (theory) in Chinese medicine is rather a discussion of and a reasoning out of the concrete and complicated relations among all the factors relevant to a particular illness course and manipulating the particular relations to effect a cure. *Zhongyi lilun* as shown in the canonical texts employs a language of imagery and metaphor (*xingxiang siwei yuyan* 形象思维语言) and allows direct access to concrete details and nuances. As such, *lilun* in the context of Chinese medicine should not be understood as referring to a coherent set of normative principles distinguished from practice. Accordingly, the canonical Chinese medical texts should not be read as norms or standardized methods by which practice is produced. Chinese medical classics, as Farquhar argues, "function more as allegorical resources for clinical thinking than as first principles."[43]

Zhongyi lilun are seen as typically embodied in the canonical texts, and learning them by heart is the way to master Chinese medical theories.[44] As I observed in clinics, a senior doctor would frequently quote a sentence or two from the medical classics to show his students the connection of his present clinical action to past knowledge and practice. Reference to such knowledge is more than just providing "symbolic anchors" to the past.[45] For many *zhongyi* doctors, those who master the medical classics well and are able to connect skillfully their own clinical actions to the practices of the past masters are considered strong in *lilun*. They believe that classical learning functions as a foundation for *zhongyi* clinical thinking.

The traditional way of becoming a *zhongyi* physician involved years of personal apprenticeship to a master physician and reading and memorizing *zhongyi* canonical texts. The importance of knowing classical texts has been always emphasized in the profession. The classic texts, such as *Neijing* (The Inner Classics), *Nanjing* 难经 (On Difficult Medical Issues), *Shanghan Lun* (Discussions of Cold Damage), and *Jinkui Yaolue* 金匮要略 (The Golden Principles), had been required readings in medical education for generations until the recent past. Although, standardized textbooks and classroom teaching are the dominant form of contemporary *zhongyi* education,[46] *Neijing* still "figures particularly prominently in contemporary teaching of the theoretical foundations of Chinese medicine, serving as a fund of ultimate explanations on which many modern writers draw."[47] For advanced students of Chinese medicine, a good knowledge of the classical medical texts is indispensable.

Compared with modern biomedical technology, *zhongyi*'s power over life and death is limited. Clinical actions therefore involve a comprehensive awareness of interdependent conditions and relations, a careful weighing of all the obvious or latent possibilities, and a grasping of the moment of opportunity for action to bring about changes. In this sense, a good clinician needs to cultivate in himself or herself an almost intuitive ability to discern subtle changes and multitude relations concerning the entire pathological condition and to flexibly deploy all the resources available for a successful intervention.[48] A diligent study of *zhongyi* classics is a time-honored way to further prepare oneself for such complicated clinical tasks. The process of learning medical classics is then a process of familiarizing oneself with the way, the style, and the language by which a particular exemplary physician demonstrated his art of medicine. Learning in this sense, similar to Hall and Ames' interpretation of "learning" (*xue* 学) in Confucian thinking, "refers to an unmediated process of becoming aware rather than a conceptually mediated knowledge of a world of objective fact."[49]

Practically, *lilun* in Chinese medicine is very much a summarized or textualized form of accumulated experience from practice (*shijian jingyan* 实践经验). It provides concrete instances and events as models and resources for organizing clinical actions. In fact, a large proportion of the publications concerning Chinese medicine throughout history have been records of medical cases (*yian* 医案), treatment formulae (*fangshu* 方书), and the personal and professional reflections (*xinde* 心得) by renowned scholar-physicians. Classic texts like these do not function to set up standards or principles for clinical practices, but to invoke, to enrich, and to inspire creativities.[50] Since the 1980s, collections of medical cases by and biographic writings of exemplary scholar-physicians of the modern time have been published in large quantity and read by new generations of physicians.

Theory or knowledge understood in this sense is not a representation of any abstract underlying truth or objective principle and therefore is not typically amenable to the absolute judgment of right or wrong. It speaks about the success of a particular moment with all its contingency and temporality. It becomes "truth" or useful knowledge when it becomes relevant to one's own moment of practice and thus becomes an integral part of the process of creating that moment. An individual physician then becomes a center or a transmitter that is both inheriting (*jicheng* 继承) and developing (*fazhan* 发展) *zhongyi* knowledge and bringing the past into the present and the future. This "distinctive" style of knowing is deeply rooted in the traditional Chinese nontranscendental and nonessentialistic worldview[51] rather than as the product of any psychologized Chinese cognitive dynamics.[52] As a medical tradition, Chinese medicine is quintessentially embodied and transmitted in the moment of clinical practice.[53] In its emphasis of personalized, textualized, and accumulated experience (*jingyan*) based on clinical practice (*shijian*), the modern world of *zhongyi* demonstrates its unity and continuity.

CONTEMPORARY CHALLENGES AND DEBATES

Zhongyi's identity in modern times is ambiguous. It is said to be ancient (*gulao* 古老), traditional (*chuantong* 传统), and as such, is aligned with the past. It is also claimed as having "scientific components" (*kexuexing* 科学性) demonstrated in its therapeutic effectiveness. Yet it does not fit comfortably into the paradigm of modern scientific medicine. "Science" (*kexue*), since the early twentieth century, has been continuously evoked to both legitimize and delegitimize *zhongyi* and to justify the *zhongyi* official policies. However, the concept of *"kexue"* (science) does not always mean the same in different historical contexts. In the early twentieth century, *kexue* meant more as the Western scientific culture—a new value system that provided an intellectual resource for China's new cultural movement aimed at overhauling the traditional Chinese culture, including Chinese medicine. From the 1950s to the 70s, *kexue* was aligned with the Maoist "dialectical materialism" (*weiwu bianzhengfa*)," referring more to the methodology or ideologically correct way in understanding "laws or patterns of the existence and development of things" (*shiwu fazhan de guilu* 事物 发展的规律) through the unity of theory and practice, to which *zhongyi* finds closer affinity than to the epistemological foundation of the modern scientific medicine.[54] In the post-Mao era, *kexue* is predominantly identified with modern Western experimental science and is viewed as the objective knowledge system, independent of any cultural, ideological, and philosophical matrix. This reading of science helped to inspire a surge of scientism that has impacted all the domains of the contemporary *zhongyi* field.

Using advanced bioscience concepts and techniques to explicate *zhongyi* theories, evaluate clinical work, and chemically analyze Chinese material medica and formulas has become mainstream in *zhongyi* research. The *zhongyi* administration at its various levels and the regulations it imposes are also increasingly modeled on their Western counterparts. In some areas, the "westernization of Chinese medicine" (*zhongyi xiyi hua* 中医西医化) is so severe that it is satirized as "running a temple as a church and having a priest guiding monks" (*siyuan dang jiaotang, shenfu guan heshang* 寺院当教堂，神父管和尚).[55"] The contemporary system of *zhongyi* education that values biosciences more than classic *zhongyi* theories as basic theoretical foundations is now faulted by many *zhongyi* scholar-physicians for producing *zhongyi* professionals who have a hard time identifying with *zhongyi* theories and methods or are merely "technologists" knowing more about treating a mouse in a laboratory setting than using *zhongyi's* way of reasoning to treat real patients (*yong zhongyi siwei fangshi* 用 中医思维方式看病).[56]

Many *zhongyi* scholars, especially senior physicians, fear that the current process of "*zhongyi* modernization" following the biomedical model will cut Chinese medicine from its cultural heritage (*wenhua chengchuan* 文化承传) and eventually render it lifeless. The various concerns for *zhongyi's* present situation and future have been discussed in a series of controversial articles under the title of "Somber Reflections on the Development of Chinese Medicine" calling for repositioning (*chongxin dingwei* 重新定位) or redefining *zhongyi* in relation to modern science.[57] This discussion has extended beyond the *zhongy;* profession and has attracted the attention of scholars from various disciplines, including scientists, historians, and philosophers, who, from the perspectives of their own specialties, advance various strategies to advocate for *zhongyi*'s independent existence and development apart from the dominance of the bio-science and its value system.[58] These strategies include: (1) detaching *kexue* (science) from the narrowly defined model of the modern experimental science and recognizing the plurality of sciences or knowledge systems; (2) aligning *zhongyi* with frontier scientific research, such as nonlinear and complexity sciences; (3) acknowledging *zhongyi*'s humanistic tradition (*renwen chuantong* 人文传统) of not separating the natural world from the human sphere and "scientific" activities from meaning systems. One thing is clear; the contending discourses of *kexue* (science) are continuing to shape the course of *zhongyi* development.

The contemporary doctors of Chinese medicine also tend to locate legitimacy of *zhongyi* in its efficacy of treatment (*liaoxiao* 疗效). For many doctors, effectiveness indicates a scientific value, as they like to say "what is effective is scientific" (*youxiaode jiushi kexuede* 有效的就是科学的). This statement finds its force in Mao's famous words in *On Practice* (*Shijian Lun* 实践论) "practice is the criterion of the truth" (*shijian shi jianyan zhenli de biaozhun* 实践是检验真理的标准), which was made into powerful political rhetoric by the post-Mao reformists in China in the early 1980s. Yet, assessing and demonstrating *zhongyi* efficacy remains a problem. Should *zhongyi* adopt the biomedical criteria and use quantifiable data based on laboratory tests to validate the claim of efficacy? It seems that *zhongyi* clinical research is moving toward such a direction. As my *zhongyi* teacher told me, "nowadays you can't just say that a therapy works; you have to show the numbers (quantitative data) and biological indications." "To establish systematic and scientific criteria for assessing *zhongyi* clinical efficacy" is recognized as one of the urgent tasks of present *zhongyi* clinical research."[59]

It is also realized that using a biomedical model to evaluate *zhongyi* therapies can lead to serious consequences, as shown by the well-known incidence of *xiao chaihu tang* (decoction of blupeuri).[60] Recent debate over the toxic side effects (*du-fu zuoyong* 毒副作用) of *zhongyao* (Chinese pharmaceutics) is another example. It raises the question: how should a toxic/side effect of a Chinese therapy be evaluated and determined? *Zhongyi* scholar-physicians, such as Yue Fengxian and Lu Guangshen, insist that when a Chinese therapy is used outside of its *zhongyi* context, for example prescribed by a biomedical doctor based on the biomedical knowledge, the unintended reaction of the medication then should not be labeled as the toxic side effect of a *zhongyao* (Chinese pharmaceutic). They argue that the use of a Chinese medical therapy has to be determined through the process of "differentiating patterns and determining therapies" (*bianzheng lunzhi* 辨证论治) as guided by *zhongyi* theories before one can talk about a toxin or side effect of that specific Chinese medical therapy.[61] Similarly, should *zhongyi* efficacy also be tested and evaluated within its own theoretical framework and therapeutic expectations? In light of the increasingly globalized *zhongyi* presence, Chinese medicine is forced to develop its own system to assess efficacy that is both accommodating to *zhongyi*'s particularity and easily accepted by the international community of medicine.

Physicians and scholars of Chinese medicine emphasize its social and cultural values in addition to its therapeutic effectiveness. They insist that *zhongyi* is a healing system that "fits Chinese national conditions" (*fuhe guoqing* 符合国情), or that *zhongyi* has "the support of the masses" (*you qunzhong jichu* 群众基础). As many Chinese medical professionals have recognized, the continuous coexistence of Chinese medicine with Western medicine in the modern scientific era in China depends on two measures, that is, to "improve" (*tigao* 提高) its efficacy and to "spread" (*puji* 普及) its knowledge. The relationship between these two aspects is very well captured in Lu's (1988) introduction to a set of popularized *zhongyi* readings:

> In order to promote Chinese medicine, it is extremely important to *tigao* (raise) the research level of professional Chinese medicine.... The central concern here is to improve clinical efficacy and to illuminate its logic by employing modern scientific methods in every possible way.... Yet, the process of *tigao* cannot be separated from the work of *puji* (popularization). Without *puji* as foundation, *tigao* is no different from building a mansion in the air.... Only after we have a large population who understand Chinese medicine, care about its future, and are willing to contribute to its cause, can we have a stable foundation to develop Chinese medicine.[62]

The official Chinese medicine, no matter how rigorous it has become, is only a limited part of the permissive *zhongyi* culture. To understand Chinese medicine, one's gaze has to go beyond the institutions of Chinese medicine and into the communities and families. Many Chinese families practice "folk versions" of *zhongyi*, using herbal remedies for minor illnesses or "as part of continuing programs of preventive home care."[63] Nowadays, in addition to keeping herbal medicines at home, families tend to store various kinds of *zhongchengyao* 中成药 (ready-made Chinese medicine in forms of pills, powder, and small balls), which are easy to understand and easy to prepare. Patients can get them without prescription in most pharmacies. Many hospitals are either associated with pharmaceutical companies or make the medications themselves. They encourage their staff to develop new medicines.[64] Experienced *zhongyi* doctors engage themselves in developing patent Chinese medicine based on classic herbal medicine formulas. On the one hand, this development makes many classic remedies readily available to people with modern lifestyles, who either do not have the time or the knowledge to prepare herbal medicines or do not care to drink bitter herbal concoctions. On the other hand, the easy access to *zhongyi* patent medicine does not come without a compromise. The flexible and individualized use of drugs based on each patient's particular condition, which is the core of a *zhongyi* therapy, gets lost in the simple matching of symptoms with the standardized ready-made medicine.

Many home medications are for treating minor disease and illness, for example, flu and cold, indigestion, and so on, but a closer look reveals that many of such therapies are meant for the complaints related to *qingzhi* disorders. Jieyu anshen chongji 解郁安神冲剂 (medicine to dispel stagnate emotions and calm the mind), a ready-made medicine developed by my *zhongyi* teacher, is meant for treating emotion-related disorders, especially "stagnation syndrome" (*yuzheng* 郁证). Even many widely used herbal "tonics" and medicinal foods, while functioning to nourish the heart and blood, are taken for the symptoms associated with the emotions.

Apparently, culture does not exist just as a way of thinking or only in philosophical reflections. It is also an embodied sense of order—persistent aesthetic values and orientations embodied in everyday bodily practices and social interactions. The Chinese cultural aesthetics that prioritize connections, transformations, and harmony manifested in the mundane practice of every day, are also the cultural sources grounding the "science" of *zhongyi* and legitimizing its practice. The next chapter offers a detailed discussion of the embodied world of Chinese culture.

III

The Chinese World of *Shenti* (Body-Person)

Phenomenologically informed medical anthropology advocates a radical role for the body as "the existential ground of culture."[1] This "anthropology of embodiment," drawing on Merleau-Ponty's phenomenology of perception and Bourdieu's theory of practice, locates culture in "the lived body" of everyday practice and directs analytical attention to the experiential aspect of culture in everyday life. The concept of "embodiment" with its intended resistance to mind/body and subject/object dichotomies in understanding human experience lends a conceptual bridge in talking about Chinese conceptions and experience of *shenti* 身体 (body-person).[2] In my analysis of *qingzhi* 情志 (emotion) disorder, I seek to situate the Chinese experience of illness and healing in the context of "embodied culture." By this, I mean the persistent and pervasive cultural values and sensibilities that are deeply rooted in bodily practices of the everyday and thus have become "natural" or habitual ways of being and doing for the local people. The idea is to make "embodied culture," or "cultural aesthetics," to follow Robert Desjarlais' use,[3] an interpretive context for understanding emotion-related disorders in the context of contemporary Chinese medicine. In this chapter, I consider how ordinary Chinese construe and experience their bodies in everyday life, what meanings and sensibilities such bodily knowledge and dispositions embody and communicate, and how these sensibilities reflect a world orientation of the people, which is also embodied in the knowledge and practice of Chinese medicine. My concern is fundamentally with meaning and the "felt quality" of cultural experiences.

This chapter centers on an exploration of the Chinese notion of "*shenti*" (routinely translated as "body" in English) and the related categories. Before we step into this Chinese world, a critical examination of the Western body in the context of Chinese culture and medicine is necessary, because when we use the English word body as a neutral analytical concept, there is always the possibility that we unconsciously read the Euro-American body into the cultural experience that is based on a different tradition of embodiment, and "necessarily import a variety of Western value orientations."[4] This problem is particularly evident in the discussions of somatization in Chinese society.

THE PROBLEM OF SOMATIZATION AND THE BODY

Chinese are widely believed to be "particularly prone to somatization."[5] A simple and familiar logic goes: psycho-emotional disorders are psychobiological entities; while cultural legitimization of emotional disorders leads to an emphasis on the psychological aspect of the disorders, the cultural stigmatization of emotional disorders leads to an emphasis on the somatic aspects of such disorders.[6] Psychologization and somatization are therefore seen as two opposite illness constructions. The former is dominant in Western industrialized society, and the latter is characteristic of more tradition-oriented society, such as China, where a "long-standing tradition of repression of emotions leads to utmost emphasis on somatic dysfunctions."[7] Seeking help with Chinese medicine for emotion-related disorders is an utmost evidence of Chinese somatization.[8]

Yet my fieldwork reveals that Chinese patients frequently relate their sufferings to emotional, psychological, and social factors in the clinics of Chinese medicine. As a matter of fact, most patients I observed in Shenjing Ke 神经 科 (the Clinic of Neuropathic Disorders) of the hospital presented emotional distress as well as bodily complaints. In my observation, Chinese patients have no problem with emotions as a source of their sufferings. They are more likely to hide from others their problem of infertility rather than their feelings of anger or sadness.[9] In some cases, instead of "somatizing" their emotional distress, Chinese patients are inclined to reject the diagnosis of an organic disease.

Ms. Wang's case is an example. Ms. Wang, in her fifties, was diagnosed as having coronary disease (guanxin bing 冠心病) in a biomedical hospital and was hospitalized for one month. Soon after she was discharged from the biomedical hospital, she went to see a senior zhongyi physician. She claimed one month of hospitalization and medication failed to cure her illness, and her symptoms became even worse. She complained about a sense of blockage (du 堵) in her heart, palpitation of her heart (xinhuang 心慌), frequent hicuups, difficulty sleeping, depletion of sweat (xuhan 虚汗) and cold extremities. She refused to accept that she had coronary disease and insisted that her illness was anger related (qide 气的). According to the zhongyi doctor, the patient suffered from liver qi stagnation (ganqi yujie 肝气郁结), obviously, a qingzhi (emotion) related disorder. For many patients, the emotion-related quality of their sufferings is precisely the reason why they come to zhongyi.[10] Zhongyi doctors accordingly see themselves as particularly strong in treating emotion-affected functional disorders, that is, qingzhi disorders.

Most zhongyi doctors simply dismiss the concept of "somatization" as irrelevant, whereas Chinese psychiatrists find themselves caught at the center of the controversy. On the one hand, they feel it important to "fit" in (jiegui 接轨) with the international community of psychiatric medicine; on the other hand, the epistemological tension between the Chinese culture of health and the modern biomedicine has to be addressed. Many of them question the general application of somatization and the related concepts to the Chinese context and suggest limiting its use.[11] For example, on the one hand, Xu argues that Chinese patients from the rural areas do not make a distinction between organic and functional disorders. On the other hand, patients from cities readily present emotional symptoms and acknowledge emotions as the source of their illness in the context of a good doctor-patient relationship.[12] For them, "bodily distress and psychic suffering are integrated and context-specific."[13] Indeed, as Yamamoto and colleagues report, instead of finding somatizing Asians versus depressive Caucasians as expected, their study of psychiatric outpatients in California reveals that symptoms of both depression and functional somatic complaints are higher among the Taiwanese than in the Caucasian comparison group.[14]

Adding complexity to this problem of somatization, Chinese verbal expressions cannot be easily categorized as somatic and psychological. For example, common symptoms presented by Chinese patients in the clinic of Chinese medicine, "blockage in the heart" (*xinli du* 心里堵) and "vexation" (*xinfan* 心烦) are experienced both somatically and psychologically. Zheng and his colleagues in their studies of styles of verbal expression of emotional and physical experience in China notice that many of the Chinese expressions do not easily fall into the categories of psychologization and somatization. They have to label the same expression, "do not want to do anything," in one place as psychological and in another place as somatic.[15] Apparently, Chinese verbal expressions of distress are mostly experiential, both emotional and somatic, neither purely psychological nor purely somatic. To categorize embodied experience according to dualistic categories can be very confusing.

In a way, this picture of somatizing Chinese represents a classic example of the Western "ethnocentrism" which, in this case, involves redefining the Chinese experience within modern Western biomedical epistemology that presupposes an essentialistic distinction between mind and body, psyche and soma, and thus psychiatric and general medical diseases. This biomedical epistemology, as Fabrega shows, postulates a "model of illness" that connects illness process and behaviors to correspondent changes in body and in mind.[16] Deviations from these norms imply either somatizing or, possibly, psychologizing. In applying this dualistic model of illness to the Chinese illness experience, researchers in fact create the very image of somatizing Chinese, which they believe to be their discovery. In fact, as illness constructions, both somatization and psychologization are products of a cultural tradition that essentializes and dichotomizes body and mind, and should only be understood in that context. They are two-way reductions of the same dualistic process.

Ironically, somatization makes much more sense in the context of modern American culture. As Pollock points out, "The fundamental bifurcation of persons in American culture into bodies and minds surely forms the cultural and historical ground for the parallel fundamental bifurcation of illnesses into the physical and the mental, and of professional medical specialties into physical medicine and psychiatry/clinical psychology."[17] Within each of these spheres of medicine, conceptions of illness as well as forms of practice tend to reflect and reproduce the basic aspect of American personhood. American patients are noticeably oriented to this dualistic principle of body and mind. As Jean Jackson shows in her study of chronic pain, patients "protest loud and clear at any hint that a given pain is 'emotional' and therefore not ultimately produced by a physical cause," because they are aware that their problems could be interpreted as "not real" or explained as mental illness or "some form of character flaw."[18] In the context of the contemporary general biomedical epistemology, a physical pain must be accompanied with a physical cause, therefore, a given pain without a physical explanation implies an illness "inauthentic if not fictive."[19] Similarly, the name of chronic fatigue syndrome (CFS) has been a topic of controversy for some time in North America. Some medical professionals feel they need to legitimatize a disorder by implying a biological basis, such as an immune dysfunction or virus infection. Patients, too, do not like the label of CFS. They insist that without a reference to a biological cause their sufferings are trivialized.[20] This type of illness experience contrasts sharply with what I observed in the clinics of Chinese medicine, where pain is simply pain experience and event, legitimate in itself, regardless of whether it is emotionally or organically caused.[21]

The cultural dualism that bifurcates the American person and medicine has a firm grounding in the Western mainstream philosophic tradition, which from its classic beginning posits inherent determinate essence as the defining principle for things.[22] Things are different by virtue of their fixed essences. The language of essentialism and the separation of the determining and the determined paved the way for the post-Cartesian framework of mind versus body, which has since permeated every aspect of the modern Western commonsense world and grounded the Western views of nature, culture, the individual, and society. They are not just "cognitive habit"[23] or a philosophic presumption; they are social values and aesthetic orientations embodied in everyday practices of the people.

Although the essentialized material body has been challenged in various postmodern writings, the fundamental dualism of mind/body "seems to be especially difficult to theorize into abandonment."[24] One reason for this tenacity lies perhaps in the English language itself. As Nancy Sheper-Hughes and Margret Lock point out, "we lack a precise vocabulary with which to deal with mind-body-society interactions and so are left suspended in hyphens, testifying to the disconnectedness of our thoughts."[25]

Whenever we use English key terms, such as *body, emotion*, or *disease*, we invoke a variety of cultural and philosophical assumptions. In the context of Chinese medicine, taking these assumptions for granted, we in fact read an ontology of substance into a more process-oriented "ontology of events,"[26] an epistemology that privileges structure and form into a more temporally organized process of transformation, a representation into more experientially oriented presentation, and a strict dualism into correlatively situated polar relations. The bodies that Chinese medicine works on and Chinese patients experience take different forms and entail a different set of vocabularies.

A SEMANTICS OF SHENTI (BODY-PERSON)

By semantics, I do not refer to an ethnosemantic analysis of the concept of *shenti*, which only deals with referential meaning. My approach, in principle, resembles Good's "semantic network analysis," which "seek(s) out for analysis the potent elements in the idiom of social interaction and explore(s) the associated words, situations and forms of experience which they condense."[27] In fact, Chinese culture is biased toward such sense of meaning in which "a term is defined non-referentially by mining relevant and yet seemingly random associations."[28]

In the contemporary Chinese language, the most commonly used expression denoting "body" or "bodily" is *shenti*, which, in fact, is composed of two root words *shen* 身 and *ti* 体. Both can be translated as "body," but the difference between *shenti* and the English word body is crucial. The English body comes from Old German *budha* meaning "tub" or "container." When body is used without further explanation and definition, it evokes in readers an image of physical, objective, or anatomic entity separate from what is spiritual and social. It requires further modification and explanation in order to convey the nondualistic experience of embodied person, such as using combined or hyphenated terms: lived body, perceiving body, mindful body, or body-mind. The English body speaks of and to a dualistic reality. In contrast, when *shenti* is used without further clarification, it implies a person or self with all the connotations of the physical, social, and mindful. As May Tung reports in her study of symbolic meanings of body in Chinese culture, with no exception, all her informants identify *shenti* with the person, the self. Some of her informants simply substituted body (*shen* 身) in her questionnaire for "the person," "the self," or simply used a personal pronoun.[29] It is the specific meaning of *shen* (regarding specifically physical, emotional, spiritual, or social aspects of a person or self) that requires further context. In other words, Chinese *shenti* is undifferentiated; its specific meaning, sometimes, requires a second character as an environment, as in the words of *shenqu* 身躯 (body trunk) or *xingti* 形体 (shape of a body).

Mark Elvin also notices that *shen* appears in most Chinese phrases that imply "person," "self," or "lifetime" in English translations. For example, *anshen* 安身—settle down in life; *shenfen* 身分—social status; *benshen* 本身—oneself; *zhongshen* 终身—to the end of one's life; *shenshi* 身世—personal history. It is for this reason that Elvin translates *shen* as "body-person."[30] The claim that due to increasing dichotomization between heart-mind and bodily emotions, the meaning of Chinese *shen* has been reduced to "body-object" seems to be problematic.[31]

Similar to *shen*, *ti* 体, the second character of *shenti*, has polysemic dimensions in use. Surely it denotes physical body, but it also extends to include meanings of form, shape, convention, style, and so on, as in *wenti* 文体 (writing style), and *zhengti* 政体 (polity). What is remarkable about *ti* is that it is often used as a verb or in a verbal phrase, meaning "to contain," "to intimate," "to implement," "to formalize," and "to understand," suggesting an agency of lived body that perceives and acts. Chinese common expressions are full of such verbs, such as *tiyan* 体验 (experience body personally) and *tihui* 体会 (understand body personally), and even *tiren* 体认 (know body personally).[32]

Susan Brownell, comparing the Chinese words *shen* and *ti*, with German *leib* and *korper*, suggests that *shen* is similar to the German concept of "*leib*" which is the subjective, experienced body, while *ti* somehow resembles the concept of "*korper*," the "alienated object body."[33] However, she seems not quite comfortable with this comparison herself and suggests that one should not take the parallels between the two Chinese and German conceptions of the body too literally because the Chinese does not exhibit strict subject-object dualism as the German does. Recognizing that in fact both *shen* and *ti* contain a subjective, experiential component, she qualifies her observation: "(N)either word has the disembodied Western sort of connotation in which a person is somehow inside the body that is experiencing life—a body that is separate from the experiencing subject."[34] If we have to make a distinction between *shen* and *ti* as bodies, we may say that *shen* implies a socially informed body-person or body-self, while *ti*, frequently used in or as a verb, emphasizes "embodying" as a process of knowing and acting. Both concepts resist dualistically positioned mind and body, subject and object. Even the modern concept of "*tiyu*" 体育 (physical education) need not be reduced to training a physical body object.[35] *Tiyu* is still very much an intense process to embody social values and ideology through a highly formalized body. In this sense, *shenti* (both *shen* and *ti*) is centrally important in Chinese social life.

Besides *shen* and *ti*, other single characters may also have the connotations of "body," for example, *xing* 形 (form, shape), *qu* 躯 (body trunk), and *shi* 尸 (corpse). In modern Chinese, they are often combined with either *shen* or *ti* to create multiple senses that indicate different states of embodiment, for example, *xingti* 形体 (body shape) and *shenqu* 身躯 (body build).

Jing 精, *Shén* 神, and *Qi* 气

Within the Western cultural dialectic going back to Plato, mind has been defined typically as a quality that transcends the body (as something that animates the body and is distinct from it). So to claim that mind is part of the body evokes contradictions. Although *jingshen*精神 is translated in English as "mind" or "spirit," it is very much part of *shenti*. *Jingshen* is formed by two root characters: *jing* 精 (concentrated basis of vitality)[37] and *shén* 神 (vitality as manifested through functional activities of mind and body as a whole). To understand the concept of "*jingshen*," we may first go to its root words: *jing* and *shén*. Both are centrally important in the Chinese conceptualization of life.

As is stated in *Neijing: Suwen* (Inner Classics: Simple Questions), "*jing* is the (concentrated) basis or root of life" (*shen zhi ben* 身之本). In contemporary Chinese medicine, it is often described as "tangible/visible life-giving substance" (*you shengming huoli de youxing wuzhi* 有生命活力的有形物质). It is implied in this statement that tangible human bodies (or any bodies), composed of muscles, skin, hair, viscera, and bones, are the results of *jing* transformation, and that *jing* as a life-giving substance is itself alive, constantly generating the new and transforming the old. *Jing* also has a narrower definition (*xiayi* 狭义), which refers to the functions of *shén* (the kidney system). This *jing* is sometimes translated as semen that is stored in the viscera of the kidney and is responsible for reproductive functions, affecting growth and aging.[38] It is therefore also called "kidney essence" (*shenjing* 肾精). In addition to reproductive functions, *shenjing* is also said to be responsible for bone growth (*zhugu* 主骨) and for producing marrow and brains (*shengsui* 生髓), therefore affecting the development of intelligence. The narrower definition of *jing* bears more clinical relevance. The symptoms of deterioration of memory, poor concentration, and mental retardation are all seen as connected to deficiency in *shenjing* (kidney essence).

Jing 精 is further differentiated as "primary *jing*" (*xiantianzhijing* 先天之精), which is inherited from one's parents (*bing yu fumu* 秉于父母) and "acquired *jing*" (*houtianzhijing* 后天之精), derived from food. Primary *jing* provides the basis for the process of transforming the energy distilled from food and is enriched and strengthened by "acquired *jing*." Chinese medical theories view *jing* and *qi* 气 (air, breath, vital energy) as the same life-giving energy. When it is concentrated, it is *jing*; when it is dispersed, it turns into *qi*. If *jing* is the nurturing aspect of this energy, *qi* is the active configurational aspect of the same energy. They come together as *jingqi* 精气 which is the basis of all forms of vitality.

However, although *jing* is described in contemporary Chinese medical discourse as "visible" (*youxing* 有形) and referred to as "substance" (*wuzhi* 物质), it cannot be isolated. Its existence can only be known and felt through its functions and effect. Healthy muscles and skin, shining hair, strong and well-formed bones, and clear memories indicate a sufficiency of *jing*. However, poorly developed bones, muscles, and intelligence may indicate insufficient *jing* in the visceral system of the kidney.

The ordinary Chinese may not be familiar with the classical or medical nuances of *jing*, nevertheless, it is part of everyday language. In lay language, '*jing*' is frequently used in combination with *li* 力 (strength, energy), both physical and mental, as something experienced, felt, and demonstrated with one's *shenti*. A person who is full of energy is said to "have plenty energy of *jing*" (*enjingli wangsheng* 精力旺盛); a person who is bogged down with endless worries may complain about "insufficient *jing*" (*jingli bugou* 精力不够); to concentrate is to "gather one's strength of *jing*" (*jizhong jingli* 集中精力); a person growing old may feel "*jing* decreasing gradually" (*jingli yitian buru yitian* 精力一天不如一天); after a strenuous task one may feel "*jing* tired out and strength used up" (*jingpi lijin* 精疲力尽).

Here, *shén* (manifested vitalities) comes in.[39] If *jing* and *qi* are the basis of life, then *shén* is the manifestation of that life. *Neijing: Lingshu* (The Inner Classics: Spiritual Pivot) says "when two *jing* (male and female *jing*) react to each other (*xiangbo* 相搏), this (confrontation) is called *shén*." In other words, *shén* is the phenomenon of life activity itself. It is typically said to be manifested in the appearance of the whole person: facial complexion and expression, especially expressions through eyes (*yanshen* 眼神), the way of talking and responding, and the movement and position of one's body. "*Shén* present" (*youshen* 有神) or "*shén* absent" (*wushen* 无神) is important information that an experienced Chinese medical doctor pays attention to when examining a patient. When *shén* is absent, even though the presented symptoms are minor, the illness is considered more serious. I noticed that while taking a patient's pulse, my *zhongyi* teacher usually spent a few quiet minutes just observing the patient before starting an extensive inquiry. He would also make some comments to bring his students' attention to any signs of *shén* of the patient. To his returning patients, he often made observations regarding their *shén*, such as "the manifestation of *shén* (*shense* 神色) looks much better this time."

Shén, in a narrow sense, may refer specifically to an individual's mental and emotional activities. This narrow sense is known as *shenzhi* 神志 (consciousness) and *qingzhi* 情志 (emotions) and is also referred to in the modern language as "*jingshen*," the combination of *jing* and *shén*. Although *jingshen* is translates as mind or "mentality," it is embedded in the cultural physiology of *jing* and *shén*, and it carries distinctive cultural semantics. One of the common complaints that Chinese present in and outside clinics is the "low level of *jingshen*" (*jingshen cha* 精神差) or "lack of *jingshen*" (*mei jingshen* 没精神). The expressions may include meanings from low physical energy and tiredness, to difficulty in concentration, poor memory, lack of interest in doing things, and depressed emotions. Lin comments that since the kidney stores *jing* and the heart governs *shén*, according to Chinese physiology, a mental disorder which is *jingshen bing* 精神病 in Chinese is literally a disorder involving the heart and the kidney.[40] The point is that *jingshen* is not perceived as opposite to *shenti* but constitutive of it.

Xin 心 (Heart-Mind) and *Nao* 脑 (Brain)

Xin commonly translated as "heart" or "heart-mind," is surely part of *shenti*. It lies literally at the heart of the Chinese understandings of person, particularly of thought and emotion.

The Chinese commonsense understanding of "the heart" is more in tune with the Chinese medicine concept of *"xin."* It is, on the one hand, understood as the most important visceral system that "governs the flow of blood in circulation vessels" (*xin zhu xuemai* 心主血脉), thus, it is responsible for coordinating the harmonious functioning of all the visceral systems of the body. On the other hand, it is the place where *shén* (spirit-vitality) is stored. *Xin* is likened to the court of a king—"the central governing visceral system where *shenming* 神明 (knowing and understanding; ethics and morals) arises."[41] *Xin* or heart-mind, though different from the anatomic organ of the heart designated usually by the term *xinzang* 心脏, is believed to be located within the chest. Its normal functioning can be felt and recognized in regular heartbeats, an even pulse, a healthy facial complexion, and also "appropriate behavior, clear mind, joyful feelings, and lucid language."[42]

Xin has social and moral significance. On the one hand, a person who is thoughtful and considerate of others and is generous and willing to help others in need is said to have a good heart-mind. On the other hand, a person is considered to have a bad heard-mind or does not even have a heart-mind if he is greedy and harbors selfish intentions toward others. Asking my friends and informants what they meant by *xin hao* (good heart-mind), I was always given concrete descriptions as to how the person behaved in relation to others. For example, a student doctor was described by others as extremely good-hearted when she volunteered to fill in on weekend duty for a colleague so this colleague could take care of an urgent family matter. Certainly, this use of the heart as moral discourse rings familiar. In English there are expressions such as a good-hearted person or a person with a golden heart. However, "heartedness" in English is generally a reference to a person's inner self. Yet Chinese do not typically understand *xin* as some fixed interior essence that defines a person but rather as a person's behaviors and attitudes toward others. The moral meaning of heart-mind lies in how a person relates himself or herself to others in the social context. "Judgment of whether a person is good or bad is therefore in terms of how this person feels and acts toward other persons."[43]

Consciousness, memorization, thinking, and forming ideas are the activities belonging to the *xin* system. The Chinese concept of "heart-mind" encompasses the functions of *nao* (brain). *Zhongyi* doctors like to say that heart-mind and brain are interconnected (*xinnao xiangtong* 心脑相通). The words *thinking* and *reflection* (*si*思), *desiring* and *imagining* (*xiang* 想), *meaning* and *intention* (*yi* 意), *desiring* and *wanting* (*yu* 慾), and planning (*lu* 虑) all have a heart radical "心"indicating that thinking, reflecting, desiring, imagining, and planning are the domains of one's heart-mind. Interestingly, *psychology* translated into Chinese becomes "studies of the patterns of heart-mind" (*xinlixue* 心理学). Nowadays, though people use both *nao* (brain) and *xin* (heart-mind) interchangeably sometimes, there is a subtle difference in meaning. The phrase I do not have the *nao* (*brain*) to do something emphasizes mental capability, but lacking the *xin* (heart-mind) to do something, the emphasis is on motivation and intention. While *nao* is reserved for more specialized discourse which is related to school or academic work and intelligence, *xin* is a more encompassing concept, appearing more in talking about the ethics, morals, intentions, desires, and emotions. A lay person's understanding of "illness of the heart" (*xinbing* 心病) may include disorders ranging from an organic heart disease to illness caused by excessive thinking and worries, worry itself, illness caused by strong desires and longings, and mental disorders.

Emotions are the domain of *xin*. The very word for "feeling" or "emotion" in Chinese is *qing* 情 which also includes *xin* as a radical, suggesting heart is also the seat of emotion. In fact, the seven emotions recognized by *zhongyi* as important elements in health, with the exception of *xi* 喜 (happy), all have *xin* as part of the characters. Chinese use *xin* to directly talk about their state of mind and emotions. The English expression I am in a bad mood in Chinese would be The circumstance/condition/sentiment of my heart is not good (*Wo xinqing buhao* 我心情不好). *Xin* appears everywhere in emotion language. Joy is literally "opening the heart" (*kaixin* 开心); happiness is "heart-sentiments flowing freely" (*xinqing shuchang* 心情舒畅); sadness is "the heart injured" (*shangxin* 伤心); compassion and affection is "heartache" (*xinteng* 心疼); and despondence is "heart-emotion depressed" (*xinqing jusang* 心情沮丧). Most Chinese emotion words bear heart radicals, such as sadness (*bei* 悲), anger (*nu* 怒), worry (*you* 忧), fear (*kong* 恐), and fright (*jing* 惊).

According to my field notes, Chinese patients who suffered *qingzhi*-related disorders tended to report symptoms directly related to *xin*. Frequently, they complained of "heart nervous" (*xinhuang* 心慌), "palpitation" (*xinji* 心悸), "heart agitation, vexation" (*xinfan* 心烦), "heart-emotion depressed" (*xinqing yayi* 心情压抑), or "heart-mind not at peace" (*xinshen buning* 心神不宁). Sometimes, a patient would attribute his or her illness to problems that also have something to do with *xin*, such as "small heart-mind" (*xinyan xiao* 心眼小) "narrow heart-edness" (*xinxiong xiazhai* 心胸狭窄), or "working one's heart-mind too much" (*tai caoxin* 太操心). *Xin* clearly occupies a centrally important role in Chinese experience of *qingzhi* disorders.

Xin grows throughout one's life but may also shrink. A patient's wife once complained about her husband, "When he gets older his heart-mind gets smaller that he cannot hold anything in his heart and constantly *xia caoxin*" 瞎操心 (operating heartmind blindly, meaning worry uselessly and unnecessarily). A person with a big heartmind is described as being able to contain and assimilate more. Heart-mind in this sense is also referred to as "heart-chest" (*xinxiong* 心胸) or even "capacity of one's abdomen" (*duliang* 肚量). My *zhongyi* teacher, Dr. Zhou, is universally praised by his students and colleagues as having "broad heart-mind" (*xinkuan* 心宽). Once a student doctor said half jokingly: "people say a prime minister's abdomen is big enough to pole a boat" (*zaixiang duli neng chengchuan* 宰相肚里能撑船), "but Dr. Zhou's abdomen is even more spacious where a warship is able to move freely." An exemplary person (*junzi* 君子) is said to have a heart-mind that is broad and open (*tandang* 坦荡); a small person (*xiaoren* 小人) entangled in his narrow heart-mind is always sullen and unhappy (*qiqi* 戚戚).

In a way, *xin* is a system of functions that forms a continuous process of being or becoming a person, involving the physiological, psychological, and sociological. The frequently quoted passage from *Neijing: Lingshu* (Inner Classics: Spiritual Pivot) describes this somato-psychic-social process of *xin* as the following:

> What responds to environment is called *xin* 心 (heart-mind).
> What *xin* brings out is called *yi* 意 (imagery)
> What *yi* stores is called *zhi* 志 (memory; memorization)
> Because of *zhi*, knowledge is reorganized.
> This is called *si* 思 (thinking; reflection).
> Because of *si*, one thinks for the future.
> This is called *lu* 虑 (strategy; plan).
> Because of *lu*, one makes decisions and takes actions.
> This is called *zhi* 智 (wise; wisdom).

Again, *yi* 意, *zhi* 志, *si* 思, *lu* 虑, and *zhi* 智 are not different things but descriptions of different phases of the same continuous process of heart-mind, where emotions and morals are not separated from thinking and perceiving. *Zhi* is *shenzhi* 神志 (consciousness) and also *qingzhi* 情志 (emotion). When much planning and calculations fail to lead to a solution, worries and anxieties arise (*bailu bu jie ze si* 百虑不解则思); on the other hand, when actions taken at the critical moment transform a dangerous situation into a favorable one, happiness arises (*fengxiong huaji ze xi* 逢凶化吉则喜). What is particular about this process-centered heart-mind physiology is not very much what Ots calls "heart-mind controlling body-emotion model,"[44] but the commitment to an unobstructed process of transformations in accordance with a given social context and natural environment.

In fact, a persistent tendency throughout Chinese intellectual culture is to see "motion and transformation" (*yundong* 运动) as generative of "the myriad things" of the world. For Zhuangzi 庄子, "the *Dao* of nature constantly transforms without stagnation, whereof myriad things are generated" (*tiandao yun er wusuoji, gu wanwu sheng* 天道运而无所积,故万物生)[45] In *Neijing: Suwen* (Inner Classics: Simple Questions), "unceasing movement leads to transformation (*dong er buyi ze bianzuo yi* 动而不已则变作矣)[46] For generations growing up reading Mao's *On Contradictions* (*Maodun Lun* 矛盾论), *yundong* is intrinsic to existence. *Dong* 动 (motion) is seen as given, while *jing* 静 (stasis, stableness) is relative and conditional, a constitutive silence or latency that marks rhythms and variations of an on-going process of *dong*. In a deeply embodied way, Chinese live in "a world of transforming effects."[47] In this world of ceaseless generative process (*shengsheng buxi* 生生不息), everything is related and yet unique (not in kind) in terms of degree (*du* 度), aspect or manifestation (*xiang* 象), situation (*qing* 情), and configuration (*shi* 势). What is essential to this world is to note "the qualities and forms of manifestations and the changing time and space relationships among them" and to look "for effective combinations that can influence developments in a desired direction."[48] Li Yiyuan also comments that Chinese throughout their lives strive to seek the best time configuration (*jishi* 吉时) in taking any important step in life.[49] Many Chinese folk religious practices involve the idea of active manipulation of timing to coordinate with auspicious cosmic time in order to exercise some control over the course of a person's life.

Then, how is *yundong* (motion/change in time) perceived and explained in the Chinese cultural world; what does this transformative cosmos mean to the people; and how does the cultural elaboration on process and change correlate to the aesthetic values and sensibilities that help shape bodily experience of everyday life and give meanings to it?

AN AESTHETICS OF *SHENTI*

I use the term *aesthetics* to indicate cultural orientations and bodily spontaneity that pattern the ways Chinese people live their lives and give meaning to their experience of *shenti* as it is nurtured (*yang* 养), cultivated (*xiu* 修), out of balance (*weihe* 违和), or healed and restored (*kangfu* 康复). An aesthetics of *shenti* 身体 is then a sense of order that is embodied through visceral experience and manifested in social interactions. My use of 'aesthetics' is influenced by Desjarlais' discussion of "aesthetic experience," in which he relates aesthetics to "the tacit leitmotivs that shape cultural construction of bodily and social interactions."[50] 'Aesthetics' in this sense refers more to cultural sensibility or orientation rather than to appreciation of artistic beauty. Illness and suffering, though lack of beauty, are still aesthetically relevant because they are "experienced and interpreted through a lens of aesthetic value."[51] An aesthetics of ordinary experience then offers a point of view to examine cultural experience as embodied, spontaneous, tacit, and also patterned, a depth that other categories of cultural analysis, such as cultural structures, models, beliefs, ideals, or rules usually do not accommodate.

The Chinese sense of order has its roots in the concept of "*dao*" (orderly processes of change) characterized by *yin-yang* dynamics.[52] *Yin-yang* is a descriptive language to talk about change and is fundamental in Chinese medical reasoning. In classical Chinese thinking, any phenomenon or process can be resolved into two opposite and complimentary aspects, that is, *yin* and *yang*. The quality of the phenomenon depends on the relationship between dynamic polarities of the *yin* aspect and *yang* aspect. For example, the daily cycle of the sun can be described in terms of waning and waxing of light and darkness. When light is maximal at noon, darkness is completely immanent. When light begins to decline after it peaks at noon, darkness begins to increase. This process of waning and waxing (*xiaozhang* 消长) continues. When darkness reaches full expression at midnight, and light is at the lowest point, the process reverses.

Nathan Sivin suggests that *yin* and *yang* "are best considered the active and latent phases of any process in space and time."[53]

The point of *yin-yang* is process, tension, and relationship of mutual constraining and generating. As summarized in modern standard textbooks of Chinese medicine, the essential meaning of *yin-yang* reasoning is about "continuity of the two opposed aspects" (*duili-tongyi* 对立统一) that are rooted in each other (*hugen* 互根), constraining each other (*xianghu zhiyue* 相互制约), and transforming into each other (*xianghu zhuanhua* 相互转化). This tension within a unity accounts for the universal dynamics of the unceasing process of generation and transformation (*shenghua* 生化). However, *yin* and *yang* are not causes of this process but descriptions of how it happens. Although abstract, they "remain rooted in concrete experience." Sivin also cautions that *yin* and *yang* are not taxonomies, and they do not sort things into fixed categories according to certain inherent essences.[54] A passage from *Neijing: Suwen* is a good illustration:

> *Yin* and *yang* are the *dao* of sky and earth (*tiandi zhidao* 天地之道), the network of myriad things, the parents of transformation and change, the root and the beginning of life-giving and life-taking (*shengsha zhi benshi* 生杀之本始), the seat of vitality and intellegence (*shenming zhi fu* 神明之府). To treat illness, one must trace this root. Thus, accumulated *yang* is sky, accumulated *yin* is earth. *Yin* is contained (*jing* 静) and *yang* restless (*zao* 躁).... When cold reaches an extreme, it gives rise to heat; when heat reaches an extreme, it gives rise to cold. Cold *qi* generates turbid (*zhuo* 浊); hot *qi* generates clear (*qing* 清). When clear *qi* (which is supposed to rise) is trapped in the lower parts of the body, it gives rise to diarrhea; when turbid *qi* (which is supposed to descend) is in the upper body, it produces swelling and fullness. This is abnormal action of *yin* and *yang*. This countermovement of *yin* and *yang* results in disorders.[55]

As shown in the passage, "the *dao* of sky and earth" mirrors the *dao* of *shenti*. In fact, the "orderly process of change" of the microcosmos of *shenti* is isomorphic to that of the macrocosmos of universe and human society. A person who has attained the *dao* coordinates and resonates with, in his/her *shenti*, the rhythmic pulse of the changes in nature. In the everyday life of ordinary Chinese, *dao* is not a philosophic or religious concept, but an aesthetic realm (*jingjie* 境界) where the coordination of a person to his or her environment has achieved bodily spontaneity. This aesthetic spontaneity of *dao* is achieved through the "mindful" process of "habituation," in concrete existence of everyday practice. *Dao* is not an objective entity of truth; it can never be independent from a particular person who practices it. For example, the *dao* of medicine (*yidao* 医道) exists only in the way that a specific doctor brings his own unique knowledge and experience and the patient's unique circumstance together and effects a healing. The spontaneity in timing; harmony in rhythms; and smooth, flowing coordination of the movements are aesthetically salient in the experience of *dao*.

In what follows, I shall outline the aesthetic values that are key to Chinese experience as they relate to illness, health, and healing.

TONG 通 (FLOWING AND CONNECTING)

Ms. Zhu went to the doctor in early April 1994. She suffered acute chest and back pain whenever she took a deep breath. Any emotional disturbance aggravated her pain. The therapeutic principle the doctor chose for treatment was "smoothing the movement of *qi* and activating the blood" (*liqi huxue* 理气活血). His prescription for the patient did not include a drug that was directly related to killing the pain. Noticing my puzzled expression, he explained that the patient's pain was related to the stagnation of her liver *qi* (*ganyu* 肝郁). In her case, the *yang qi* was gathered and trapped (*yuzhi* 郁滞) within the chest that blocked the passage of normal movement of *qi*. He quoted the Chinese medical wisdom that "when the circulation (of *qi*) is blocked, pain arises, when the passage is open, pain disappears" (*butong ze tong, tong ze butong* 不通则痛, 通则不痛). The idea of his treatment was to get *qi* moving again. Once that was accomplished, the patient's pain would disappear automatically. The association of the experience of pain (*tong* 痛) to the blockage (*butong* 不通) of *qi* is a marked clinical manifestation of Chinese medical disorders. Pain then has a culturally distinctive meaning and pattern of a blocked circulation. The experience is certainly informed by a culturally cultivated sense of order: a continuous process that should be well coordinated at all the levels of human existence—the cosmic, social, personal, and the bodily.

Chinese people are oriented to the sense of a smoothly flowing process, which is characterized by such images as *tong* (open, through, extending, connecting, continuing, and flowing), *huo* 活 (alive, active, and flexible), or *shun* 顺 (unobstructed, smooth). These images are positively valued by Chinese in their *body* as well as in their social world.[56] Negative images opposite to *tong, huo,* and *shun* are blockage, obstruction, stagnation, death, and lifelessness.

This aesthetic orientation of the everyday is also played out in Chinese social life. The Chinese are known for placing great emphasis on cultivating social networks (*guanxi* 关系).[57] *Guanxi* networks have acquired "personal circulation vessels" (*renmai* 人脉) as in the expression of *Renmai fengpei* 人脉丰沛, meaning, literally, "having rich and numerous personal circulation vessels." These circulation networks are developed to ensure "personal or group survival and development."[58] The image of the expression is physiological. Similar values applied to physiological circulation are also oriented to in social circulations. Persons who are good at cultivating networks are described as having many/flexible channels (*luzi duo/huo* 路子多/活). The image for those who do not cultivate *guanxi* is death (*si* 死). In some areas, those who are disadvantaged in establishing networks are described as "dead doors" (*si menzi* 死门子) that lead to nowhere.[59] The aesthetic values shown in *tong, huo,* or *shun* also guide Chinese people in creating and developing social relationships through all forms of reciprocity of giving and taking.

The sense of obstruction or disconnection (*butong, bushun*) in the social world can be simultaneously experienced bodily and emotionally. A patient, who was a computer technician, told me that his life was not going anywhere no matter how hard he tried, as if he had reached a wall and could never get over. He explained that most of his classmates who had graduated from college at the same time as he were either promoted to higher positions, found a better job, or went abroad. He, a good student at school, was now left behind. He could not keep up with the pace of others. Noticeably, others are the reference points for a person to assess how well he or she "moves" in the social world. Feelings of being left behind can be overwhelming. He used to think that as long as he worked hard he could get ahead. But now he devotes almost all his waking hours to his studies and work, and the result was the opposite. His memory seems weak, and he can hardly concentrate on his work, as if the functions of his whole *shenti* slowed down, leading to a slow reaction (*fanying man* 反应慢), low vitality level (*jingshen cha* 精神差), nervous heart beating (*xinhuang* 心慌); feeling of closure/pressure in the chest (*xiongmen* 胸闷), and heart-emotion depressed (*xingqing yayi* 心情压抑). According to the Chinese doctor's diagnosis, this patient also suffered from *ganyu* (stagnation of *qi* in the liver system).

Chinese medicine has numerous words describing all kinds of blockages and stasis in subtle differentiations. *Yu* 郁 is mainly stagnation of *qi*, which is invisible (*wuxing* 无形) and which is closely related to disordered emotions;[60] *yu* 瘀 is stasis of tangible (*youxing* 有形) fluids, such as blood; *zhi* 滞 is sluggish movement (of *qi*); *ji* 积 is accumulation of something (*shiji* 食积 is accumulation of food); *jie* 结 is coagulation, sometimes in the form of a lump; *zu* 阻 is obstruction or blockage of the circulation passages. These physiological dysfunctions are often experienced by Chinese patients as *tong* 痛 (pain), *du* 堵 (blockage usually in heart or in one's throat), *men* 闷 (stuffiness in the chest), and *zhangman* 胀满 (fullness in chest area). *Yu* (stagnation/blockage) occupies such an important role in the clinical manifestation of Chinese medicine that some famous doctors in the history of Chinese medicine insist that *yu* is the single most important factor that results in medical disorders.[61]

If a phenomenology of depression is universally characterized by "soul loss" (feeling of emptiness),[62] then the Chinese experience of *yu* disorders is strikingly different phenomenologically, though some of the symptoms may appear familiar. In fact, emptiness (*kong* 空 or *xu* 虚) is not always a negative feeling. *Kong* or *xu* can be positive in the Daoist sense of a "dissolved self" (*wuwo* 无我) that by virtue of its "emptiness" permeates everywhere. In modern everyday Chinese, the image of emptiness is also used to convey the sense of open-mindedness or humbleness. A tolerant and openminded person is "having an inside as empty or spacious as a valley" (*xuhuai-ruogu* 虚怀若谷). A morally mature person is able to "make room in oneself to accommodate others" (*xuji-dairen* 虚己待人). The quality of "emptying one's heart" (*xuxin* 虚心), meaning modesty or readiness in opening oneself to see other people's point of view, is a widely advocated virtue in a person. As for experience of feelings, *kong* 空 as in "empty and quiet" (*kongji* 空寂) and *xu* 虚 as in "empty and peaceful" (*xujing* 虚静) describe an aesthetically pleasant meditative state of peacefulness and wholeness. The Chinese experience of *qingzhi* disorders is largely characterized by *yu* (stagnation), a sense of *butong* (almost opposite to emptiness)—obstruction and blockage to orderly motions and extensions. The main form of *qingzhi* disorders is *yuzheng* (illness of *qi* stagnation). The character *yu* appears in the Chinese translation of the psychiatric term of depression *yiyu* 抑郁. It is also part of the word *youyu* 忧郁, which, in modern Chinese, means sadness and melancholy.[63] Revealingly, the Chinese feelings of unhappiness and sadness are associated with the experience of stagnation and blockage in one's existential world. Happiness is associated with the experience of unblocked and unimpeded flowing as shown in the expression of "freely stretching and flowing of heart-mind" (*xinqing-shuchang* 心情舒畅).

DU 度 (DEGREE/POSITION AND MODERATION)

In the Chinese aesthetic world, a myriad of things are connected in an unceasing process of changes and transformations and are differentiated according to "numerous positions on the continuum" of the process between extremes,[64] such that things are recognized as different according to their *du*, the degree or position, rather than solely or mainly to any fixed essence. *Du* is therefore centrally important in understanding Chinese experience.

For example, mental illness in Chinese is *jingshen bing* 精神病, but not all the psychogenic disorders are labeled as *jingshen bing*. In the Chinese understanding, psychological or emotional disorders, only when they come to a certain degree, can be labeled as *jingshen bing*. As Lee and Wang report in their Hong Kong studies, neurasthenia is perceived to be psychogenic by Hong Kong Chinese students, however, they also insist it is not a mental illness. At the same time they agree that when neurasthenia becomes severe, it may lead to schizophrenia, which then becomes a mental illness.[65] Psychiatrists working with Chinese culture mostly interpret this "contradiction" as caused by stigmatization of mental illness in Chinese society. Surely, severe mental illness may be socially stigmatized, yet this is not a phenomenon unique to Chinese culture. It is also commonly known that in Western society, mental illnesses are stigmatized socially if not medically.[66] In China, *jingshen bing*, in commonsensical language, almost always refers to relatively severe psychiatric disorders that upset the normal social functions of a person and create disturbance to the family and the community. General emotion-related disorders are perceived as some form of "body-heart disorders" (*shenxin jibing* 身心疾病) or recently "subhealth conditions" (*ya jiankang zhuangtai* 亚健康状态), which are viewed as benign and highly reversible. Similarly, the Chinese translation of major depression is *"zhongxing yiyuzheng"* 重型抑郁证 (severe depression), which translates a typological concept into a concept of degree. This "translation difficulty," Lee suspects, might account partially for miscommunication between Chinese psychiatrists and their Western counterparts and might also account for differential diagnosis of major depression in China.[67]

Western students easily miss the centrality of *du* 度 (degree, tensity, quantity) in Chinese experience. The interpretation that since excessive emotion is seen as detrimental to health, emotions or an overly demonstrative expression of emotions are therefore highly stigmatized. This is echoed in many major studies of emotion and emotional disorders in Chinese society.[68] For example, Ots argues that in Chinese medicine: "According to the theory of systematic correspondence (*wu xing xueshuo*) these emotions, when in excess, hurt their corresponding viscera as well as the encompassing heart-mind. Emotional behavior, therefore, is heavily stigmatized."[69] From the *zhongyi* point of view, such logic is problematic. The concept of *"guodu"* 过度 (surpassing the *du*, excessive) to Chinese is itself valid in defining and establishing a situation. Emotions that surpass the *du* are sufficiently different in significance from the emotions within the *du*. In addition, emotions are seldom talked about and experienced as abstract concepts, but always in relation to concrete social situations that also specify appropriate *du* of actions. In other words, it is not "emotion," but the excess defined in concrete social contexts with certain social and bodily effects that is harmful to one's health. My impression is that it is almost "natural" for Western-trained scholars to see excessive as merely an adjective, a qualifier. It is emotion, which is essentialistically determined, that defines and counts. The sense of *du* gets lost when excess of emotion is interpreted as simply emotion or emotional expressions or behavior. In addition, excess not just in emotion but in almost everything else is viewed negatively by the Chinese: for example, excess in thinking may be harmful to one's heart and spleen *qi* (*silu guodu shang xinpi* 思虑过度伤心脾), and excess in eating and drinking hurts one's spleen and stomach systems (*yinshi guodu shang piwei* 饮食过度伤脾胃). It would be absurd therefore to assert that Chinese culture also stigmatizes thinking and eating.

Appropriate sense of *du* is also a form of *de* 德 (virtue, morals), the heart of Confucian doctrine of *zhongyong* 中庸 (the mean) which advocates a social political order that does "not lean to any one side" (*bupian buyi* 不偏不倚) and is "neither excessive nor insufficient" (*wu guo buji* 无过不及). This moral sense of *du* is well expressed in Confucius's own words: "Grieve but not to the extent of injury, enjoy but not to the extent of excess" (*ai er bu shang, le er bu yin* 哀而不伤, 乐而不淫). One of the major tasks of "cultivating one's body-person" (*xiushen* 修身) is to develop the spontaneity of *du* and the sensibility of harmony and moderation (*zhonghe* 中和). A mature person (an adult) is expected to demonstrate the sensibility of *du*, knowing the boundaries (*fencun* 分寸) (literally decimeters and inches) and limits (*jindui* 进退) (literally advance and retreat). Both excess (*guo* 过) and insufficient (*buji* 不及) are considered undesirable. It is a cliché among Chinese that truth, taken a step further, becomes false. Many commonly used phrases convey this cultural sensibility of *du*, such as "stop when it is right" (*shike'erzhi* 适可而止) or right to the appropriate point (*qiadao haochu* 恰到好处).

The sense of *du* is embodied, acquired, and developed in concrete everyday existence through the ways the Chinese interact with each other, care for their young and old, enjoy a piece of music, or cook a bowl of soup. *Du* is not a normative concept or a fixed standard by which one determines if a behavior is excessive or not. Therefore, assuming overt expression of emotion or emotional behavior is meant by Chinese as excessive and therefore is highly disvalued and cautiously guarded against is a misinterpretation. *Du* is rather an experiential concept, which can only be sensed and felt in concrete human situations. Excess or not is not determined by standard measurement but is contingent on the actual circumstances and effects.[70] This is common sense to Chinese medical doctors. Each person is a unique unity of psycho-physical dispositions (*xing* 性) and socioenvironmental conditions, such that for one person at one time and place, it is normal, and for another person or at another time and place, it may be excessive. In simple words, a doctor said to me, "I may eat as many pieces of cold watermelon as I like without feeling any discomfort. You may have a stomachache or diarrhea after just having two pieces, so in your particular case, one piece is right to the *du* and two pieces are excessive."

Excess (surpassing the *du*) cannot be judged independently from its effect. Asking my Chinese friends to define emotional excess, instead of getting abstract normative answers, I was offered various emotional scenarios. For instance, the story of Fan Jin passing the provincial imperial examination was mentioned to show excess in the emotion of joy. In the story, when Fan Jin heard that he had passed the provincial imperial examination after many years' disappointment, he was so overjoyed that he suddenly went crazy. Similarly, when Potter asked her informants about emotional excess, she was told about an old woman who, after the death of her child, cried so much that she became blind.[71] Excess and effect mutually entail each other in this sense. If excessive thinking and worrying (*silu guodu* 思虑过度) "causes" (the Chinese sense here is closer to "contributes to") the syndrome of "heart-yin deficiency" (*xinyin buzu* 心阴不足) characterized by symptoms of "hot sensation in five-centers" (*wuxin fanre* 五心烦热), "disturbed heart-mind" (*xinshen buning* 心神不宁), "heart vexation" (*xinfan* 心烦), and "insomnia" (*shimian* 失眠), these symptoms may also indicate an excess in thinking and worrying.

Since *du* is not a normative concept, it should not be seen as an external constraint forced on members of the society from the outside and leading to "repression and suppression of emotions." It is rather an aesthetic value that people are oriented to and engaged with in their daily lives. It functions constitutively and immanently within the order of everyday life itself.

HE 和 (HARMONY)

The concern of harmony (*he* 和 or *hexie* 和谐) is evident everywhere in Chinese culture from highly ritualized ceremonial perfomance and structured social relations to mundane practices of the everyday. Some scholars believe that "seeking balance and harmony" (*zhizhonghe* 致中和) has been an enduring cultural sensibility in Chinese tradition that guides how Chinese, including well-cultivated elites and rudimentally educated laborers and peasants as well, live their lives.[72] The common expressions of today, such as "harmony brings wealth" (*heqi shengcai* 和气生财) and "all flourishing when there is harmony at home" (*jiahe wanshixing* 家和万事兴) still echo the passage in the classic *Zhongyong* 中庸 (*The Doctrine of the Mean*): "When harmony is reached, the sky and the earth follow their proper routes and myriad things flourish in life" (*Zhi zhonghe, tiandi wei yan, wanwu yu yan* 致中和, 天地位焉, 万物育焉). Ordinary Chinese are often found quoting the proverb from the *Analects*: "harmony is most valuable" (*heweigui* 和为贵) when persuading others to resolve conflicts or explaining their own behaviors of reconciliation. The origin of the saying can be traced back to the statement "the most valuable function of propriety is to ensure harmony (*lizhiyong, heweigui* 礼之用和为贵) in *Lunyu* 论语 (*The Analects: 1*) more than two thousand years ago. The recent discussions of "culture of harmony" (*hehe wenhua* 和合文化) in China stress that "*he*" is a persistent and most commonly accepted cultural value throughout Chinese history.[73]

According to Li, the overall sense of harmony for Chinese depends on harmonious relationships at three levels: harmony at the level of natural environment, harmony at the level of body-person (*shenti*), and harmony of social relations (both interpersonal and to the spiritual world).[74] Since an aesthetics of harmony is embodied, disharmony at any of the three levels upsets the bodily sense of order. Therefore, *he* as a key aesthetic value is quintessentially reflected in Chinese medicine, an art of health and healing. *Zhongyi* sometimes is actually referred to as "medicine of harmony" (*zhonghe zhi yi* 中和之医). As is stated in *Neijing*, "when *qi* and *blood* move in harmony, no illness will arise" (*qixue chonghe, baibing bu sheng* 气血冲和百病不生). So falling ill is the "body-person falling out of harmony" (*shenti weihe* 身体违和). In fact, many Chinese medical disorders can be summarized simply as "out of harmony" (*buhe* 不和) or "out of balance" (*butiao* 不调). Many times, the doctors I observed simply explained to their patients that they suffered "*yin* and *yang* not in harmony" (*yinyang buhe* 阴阳不和) "spleen and stomach *qi* not in harmony" (*piwei buhe* 脾胃不和), or "*qi* and blood out of balance" (*qixue butiao* 气血不调) so that the patients could grasp basic ideas without the doctors using too much *zhongyi* jargon.

According to Chinese medical reasoning, "a human body-person resonates with the way of sky and earth" (*ren yu tiandi xiangying* 人与天地相应). The movement of *qi and* blood and the functions of the visceral systems and other bodily systems may demonstrate different characteristics in accordance with the changes of "sky and earth." A person is encouraged to anticipate the changes and adapt one's behavior to the changes. The importance of harmony of a person in relation to the changes of the macroenvironments, such as the changes of seasons, weather, temperature, and moisture during the day or the year is stressed in all kinds of popular publications on "cultivating life" (*yangsheng* 养生).

He (harmony) is often cited as the most important factor leading to social success and achievement. Three elements are considered by Chinese as important in virtually any kind of success. These are right time (*tianshi* 天时), advantageous position (*dili* 地利), and harmonious interpersonal relationship (*renhe* 人和). In comparison, harmonious interpersonal relationship is deemed more important than the other two elements, as shown in the still popular expression quoted from *Mencius* that "the right time yields to advantageous position; advantageous position yields to harmonious interpersonal relationship" (*tianshi buru dili, dili buru renhe* 天时不如地利, 地利不如人和). The cultural aesthetics of *renhe* (harmonious interpersonal relationship) finds its full expression in Chinese family ethics that guide the way the family members care for and interact with each other according to their places within the family. The harmonious family also includes a vertical dimension. This concern for harmonious family relationships extends to the deceased members of the family, that is, the spiritual world.[75] Apparently, the cultural sense of harmony (*he*) is also at work when Chinese take care of their ancestors' tombs, and offer foods and burn paper money to their ancestors. It is still a common practice in many rural areas that family members, believing in a harmonious reciprocity with one's ancestors, pay respect to their ancestors following a personal success such as passing a college entrance examination. Here, the Chinese spiritual world is connected with the present world. This is also related to the Chinese sensibility of *tong* (connection and flowing) discussed above. For the Chinese, harmony presupposes a healthy process of connecting and extending.

It is also important that the cultural aesthetics of *renhe* (harmonious interpersonal relations) extend beyond one's immediate circle of family members and relatives through extensive networks of "human emotions" (*renqing* 人情) created and maintained diligently by all forms of social exchanges, of gifts, labor, services, respect, and so on.[76] Li points out that the ultimate goal of Chinese exchange relationship is to seek harmony and balance in the social world, that resonates harmoniously with the macrocosmos of nature and the microcosmos of body-person.[77]

Western scholars often tend to associate an emphasis on harmony with repression or suppression of emotions in Chinese social life, as if there is an intrinsic conflict between harmony and emotions. Yet, if we give the Chinese concept of harmony, "*he*," a close examination, we can see that *he* does not mean forcing a conformity by appealing to a single existing standard. According to the *Zhongyong* 中庸 (*The Doctrine of the Mean*), "latent emotions of happiness, anger, sadness, and joy are called neutral (*zhong* 中); when active and yet appropriate (*zhongjie* 中节), they are called harmony (*he*)." Harmony defined here is related to the Chinese sense of *du* (degree, extent, position) discussed previously. *Zhongjie* literally means "hit the rhythm," or "right to the mark" conveys the sense of *du* that is neither excessive nor insufficient (*wu guo buji* 无过不及). In other words, in a dynamic interactive environment, harmony is brought out when each particular unfolds itself in its unique way and to an appropriate *du* such that "each shines more brilliantly in the other's company" (*xiangde-yizhang* 相得益彰). In fact, early Chinese thinkers had already made a clear distinction between the concept of harmony (*he*) and that of "sameness and conformity" (*tong* 同). For example, in Guo Yu: Zheng Yu 国语: 郑语 (compiled during the Easten Zhou period 475 BC–221 BC), it is stated that "to complement one thing with a different thing is called harmony, with which things flourish and join each other; yet to strengthen one thing by adding the same thing (which is called conformity), brings an end to everything."[78] In the Chinese sense, harmony presupposes diversity, differentiation, and confrontation. Similarly, Ames and Hall translate *he* as "attuning": "combining and blending of two or more ingredients in a harmonious whole with benefit and enhancement that maximizes the possibilities of all without sacrificing their separate and particular identity."[79]

As shown above, Chinese people in their everyday lives are, explicitly or tacitly, oriented to a set of cultural aesthetic values. The aesthetic sensibilities are evident in their way of "making the world," in their experience of illness when the world is "unmade" by blocked circulations (*butong*), lack of moderation (*shidu*), or loss of harmony (*weihe*), and in the process of "remaking their world" through healing, known also in Chinese medicine as attuning (*tiao* 调). Emotions, as viewed from the perspective of Chinese medicine, are centrally important to this process of making and unmaking the world of body-person. The following chapter focuses on the Chinese concept of "emotions" and explores the cultural world of emotional meanings as they relate to illness and healings.

IV

Contextualizing *Qingzhi* 情志 (Emotions)

An ethnographic study on illness and health that addresses socioculturally constituted "body-person" necessarily entails a translation of a cultural world of
emotional meanings. This is particularly relevant to our understanding of the
disorders that are perceived locally as "emotion-related," such as *qingzhi* 情志
disorders in Chinese medicine. Two recent lines in anthropological thinking
of emotion lend complementary perspectives to this enquiry. The sociocultural
construction approach advocated and practiced by anthropologists such as Abu-
Lughod, Lutz, and White, focuses typically on emotions as discursive (meaning
making) social practice,[1] while the phenomenologically inspired approach adopted by such anthropologists as Cosdas, Desjaleis, Lock and Sheper-Hughes
pays ultimate attention to the felt or embodied quality of emotional experience.[2]
Seeing *qingzhi* and disordered *qingzhi* as an interactive social phenomenon and
embodied experience informed with the cultural sensibilities of *tong* 通 (flowing, extending), *du* 度 (degree, position, intensity), and *he* 和 (harmony), this
chapter explores the sociocultural and ethnomedical contexts where *qingzhi*
and disordered *qingzhi* are formulated, talked about, and experienced.

UNRAVELING *QING* 情 (EMOTION)

The studies that theorize the Chinese experience of emotions are marked by
their contradictory observations and rivaling interpretations. Arthur Kleinman,
for example, in his works about the Chinese experience of illness and health,
describes emotion-tacit Chinese who through socialization have learned that
personal affects, especially negative or disphoric emotions, should not be openly
expressed. He generalizes that in Chinese society negative emotions such as depression, sadness, and irritability are suppressed and not to be revealed outside
one's family.[3] Ots also argues that Chinese culture stigmatizes emotional behaviors and that open expression of emotion is devalued and carefully guarded
against.[4] However, Potter and Potter contend that such a generalization does
not conform to the observed social reality. According to Potters' observation in

a village in Guangdong, villagers are actually emotionally expressive in every sense including the emotions that could be listed as dysphoric, strong, and negative or even hostile. They then argue that Chinese emotions are natural phenomena lacking important social and symbolic significance "for the maintenance and perpetuation of social relationships."[5] Andrew Kipnis, drawing on his own ethnographic experience in the countryside of Shandong, takes issue with Potter and Potter. He argues that Chinese emotion is indeed a social performance through which social relationship is established and maintained. One of the most obvious points of evidence he mentions is that during the cultural revolution, the cross-class crying at funerals was banned because ritual crying at a funeral, a mode of emotional expression, was perceived as establishing and consolidating a social relationship, and any such cross-class demonstration of relationship was deemed politically incorrect at the time. Kipnis argues if it were true that Chinese emotion, as Potter and Potter have argued, did not have any formal social significance, cross-class crying at funerals would not have been a concern at all.[6]

These observations, seemingly inconsistent, do have a contribution to make. The cultural sensibility of shame and face-saving does play its role in the way Chinese express and experience their emotions.[7] In clinical interactions, doctors usually do not explicitly pursue sensitive personal information, but rather rely on their own developed sensitivity to ascertain the problems. Yet emotions are expressed openly everywhere, sometimes very forcefully. For example, Chinese are notorious for their open displays of anger on buses. Martin Schoenhals observed that every day or two, he encountered an argument or a fight on the street or on the bus.[8] An American friend also told me that he was surprised to see how ordinary Chinese could openly display their strong emotions toward authoritative figures. He referred to an incident he saw in Beijing where a cyclist, after being stopped by a policeman, yelled angrily at the policeman and drew a crowd of onlookers. I personally observed at numerous times in the clinics that patients cried openly in front of doctors and other patients while talking about their illness, frustrations, and sadness. Of course, such expressiveness does not logically lead to the conclusion that Chinese emotion has no formal social significance. On the contrary, expressing emotion is always open to social and moral interpretations and judgment. Emotions, such as "moral indignation" (yifen 义愤) and "public indignation" (gongfen 公愤) are used frequently to justify social actions. I agree with Schoenhals who suggests, in his ethnographic study of a Chinese middle school, that expression of emotions in Chinese society is highly contextualized and that in certain social contexts expressiveness and aggression are tolerated, sanctioned, and even expected.[9] We may also say that certain emotions or certain ways of doing emotions are called for in certain contexts or within certain structural relationships. The absence of them invites interpretations and judgment, too. In other words, a good understanding of the Chinese experience of emotion lies in the culturally informed sensitivity to contexts, given that the Chinese cultural tradition in general is interested more in process and events rather than in essence and agency.[10]

If we take "emotion inside out" as Geoffrey White suggests, the understanding of emotion, then, does not require a commitment to any particular ontology of emotions, but involves "the study of meaning making practices of persons engaged in ordinary talk and interactions."[11] At the same time, we need to see how emotion is conceptualized within the culture and how a particular emotion "fits into the systematic world view, language, and way of life of the society."[12] What is involved is "a tracing out and unraveling of the relationships and conditions of the phenomenon's context, and its multiple correlations."[13] In other words, a more informative way to understand the meaning of Chinese emotion is to map out a network of meanings, situations, experience, and events that typically associate with "*qing*" (emotion). Again, this approach is inspired by Byron Good's model of semantic network analysis, which fits well in the enduring Chinese mode of knowing characterized by the "one evoking many" model.[14] It is particularly relevant to how *zhongyi* works, where certain symptoms, experiences, and situations are viewed as typically associated with one another to form a cluster or pattern known as "syndrome cluster or pattern" (*zhenghouqun* 症候群). One obvious difference between an experienced doctor and an inexperienced one in clinical work, according to my *zhongyi* teacher, is that an experienced doctor is familiar with *zhenghou qun* and thus is more efficient in mapping out the illness situations and tracing the roots of the problem. Similarly, understanding of *qingzhi* will benefit from mapping out a network of associated meanings and events of "*qing*" and tracing the meaning to its root.

Like many other key terms in the Chinese language, *qing* hardly translates unambiguously. *Li Ji* 礼记 (The Book of Rituals ca. 465–450 BCE) defines '*qing*' as the human feelings of "joy, anger, sadness, fear, like, dislike, and desire—the seven (abilities) acquired (by human beings) without the deliberate effort of learning." Xunzi also sees *qing* as a person's natural tendency (*xing* 性) of "likes and dislikes, joy, anger, and sadness."[15] Dong Zhongshu, the Confucian scholar of the early Han dynasty, refers to *qing* as "human capacity of desiring, wanting, and motivating" (*ren zhi yu* 人之欲). The definition of *qing* that has more or less continued up to today stresses the interaction of human beings with their environment. For example, Han Yu of the Tang dynasty writes, "*Qing* arises when (a person) comes into contact with the world" (*qingyezhe, jieyuwu er sheng* 情也者, 接于物而生).[16] *Qing* seems to be broader than emotive states and "includes all reality inputs"[17] or perhaps all reality configurations. *Qing*, therefore, is "*ganqing,* 感情" (sentiments or feelings, emotional attachment), "*aiqing* 爱情" (good feelings and love between couples), and "*qingyu* 情欲"—(sensual desires). *Qing* is also "*qingmian* 情面" (social face), "*renqing* 人情" (social obligation and ethics, a social network), "*qingli* 情理" (commonsense, reasons), and "*qingkuang* 情况" or "*qingxing* 情形" (situations, circumstances, or reality). *Qing* presupposes participation in social relations and interactions. Indeed, as Solomon comments, one cannot feel any of the emotions, such as love, anger, sadness, shame, without engaging others in one's experience.[18] Importantly, *qing* is a relational and situational concept. Chinese tend not to conceptualize emotions as pure inner feelings separated from concrete situations. Emotions are not talked about and experienced as abstract concepts but in relation to particular social situations. *Qing*, therefore, is correlated with reason or rationality (*li* 理), speech or language (*yan* 言), behavior or action (*xing* 行), and appropriateness (*yi* 义).

Qing as *Sensibility of Face*

The English expression *hurting somebody's feelings* may simply translate as "injuring somebody's face" (*shang mianzi* 伤面子) in Chinese. As many scholars have previously pointed out, the concept of "face" is central to the Chinese experience and is an important mechanism of social control.[19] In addition, face is frequently expressed and experienced in terms of emotions.

The Chinese sense of face is recognized as having two aspects: *mianzi* 面子 (social face) and *lian* 脸 (moral face).[20] *Mianzi* is talked about in terms of social status and prestige. It is the personal merit recognized by the public. This type of face is constantly under public scrutiny and subject to society's evaluations. Logically, some have bigger *mianzi* than others. Those who are more educated and cultured (*you wenhua* 有文化), those who are distinctively recognized, and those who have higher social status, have bigger *mianzi* and consequently bear the burden of living up to higher expectations. They are subject more easily to public humiliation and hence to the experience of losing face (*diu mianzi* 丢面子) which can be intensely emotional. I personally experienced such an incident when I accidentally parked my bicycle along with several other bicycles in an area where bicycle parking was not allowed. After I showed my identification card, the old guard deliberately pointed out for everybody to hear that with my background as a teacher what example I was setting for my students if I could not follow the rules myself. This retired worker, without his red band around his left arm, would be perfectly negligible. But with his indignant look and raised voice accusing somebody well educated, he suddenly gained social face and became more important. Moreover, I was made to lose face and to feel totally humiliated. Under the circumstances, the only thing for me to do was to leave the scene as quickly as possible. To argue was to lose face even more. The experience of losing face can be very painful.

The sense of *mianzi* is not just something superficial or skin deep. It is said to have something to do with one's "heart of self-respect" (*zizunxin* 自尊心). Those who have a strong sense of self-respect are more sensitive to *mianzi*. *Lian* 脸, is used in talking about moral and ethical sensibility. A person whose conduct trespasses moral codes loses his or her "moral face" (*dui lian* 丢脸), which is considered more serious. "Do not want moral face" (*buyao lian* 不要脸) is one of the most insulting remarks one can make, implying that the person "has laid aside all claims to be a person."[21] The sense of *lian* depends on the sense of shame (*xiuchi xin* 羞耻心), a painful feeling similar to guilt.

Some scholars consider that the sense of *lian*, unlike the sense of *mianzi*, which depends on external sanction of behaviors, functions as an "internal moral restraint."[22] However, *mianzi* and *lian* are not two totally separate phenomena. Both involve social norms and a personal sense of pride and shame. *Mianzi* and *lian* are rather the same process of being a person seen or talked about from different points of view. *Mianzi* is seen from the outside extending to the inside, while *lian* is seen and experienced from the inside extending outside. In the experience of a real life situation "moral face" and "social face" are integrated. For this reason I prefer to use *lian-mian* 脸面 (face), except in the situations where one meaning is overwhelmingly dominant, to indicate the complexity of the Chinese concept of face.

Face is an integrative part of becoming a person, and every mature Chinese person (adult) is expected to be sensitive to face. Sometimes talking about face is another way of talking about "feelings." However, face is more a dynamic phenomenon in Chinese social life that one can lose, gain, give, protect, or even buy. In fact, it is fair to say that Chinese in everyday life engage themselves actively in the process of a "face economy."[23] Compared to other aspects of face, the loss of face or a threatened loss of face is more experienced and talked about in terms of emotions. Schoenhals argues that loss of face is "fundamentally an emotional reaction (usually temporary) of a person who failed to live up to others expectations."[24] A patient informant clearly related his illness to his feeling of loss of face. He told me that he used to be a very good student in college, and everybody thought he was smart. His company spent money sending him to Japan for training and made him the director of his section. He was overcome by the burden of having to live up to his reputation. He was worried that he might be found to be incompetent in his position and unworthy of his reputation. He therefore spent all his energy trying to stay ahead of his colleagues. Now with an exhausted body-heart (*shenxin* 身心), he thought that the colleagues who came to the company much later could perform better work than he did. "Now everybody knows I am not that smart after all," he said. This, to him, was very face threatening. Yet the intensity of a person's experience of loss of face is not necessarily coordinated with the public's evaluations. Sometimes with little actual public display, a person may feel an intense loss of face. It depends more on a person's perception of the public's response or on how much a person is oriented to social norms and moral codes. An informant talked about his feelings of guilt/shame (*kuijiu* 愧疚) and incompetence (*wuneng* 无能) when he, the first son of the family, had to delay his aging mother's coming to live with his family because he did not have enough space in his one-bedroom apartment. He kept telling his mother he was going to be assigned a bigger apartment soon, but each time he was disappointed. He became suicidal, feeling that he had failed both his social and moral obligations.

Like the Chinese concept of "person," face can extend to include groups with which one is identified. Literally, one can lose one's parents' face (*diu fumu de lian* 丢父母的脸), one's family's face (*diu jiaren de lian* 丢家人的脸), and even lose one's country's face (*dui guojia de lian* 丢国家的脸). Chinese soci-ety is connected in such an extensive way that everybody can potentially lose everybody else's face. A misbehaving child may lose her parents' face, and an incompetent or immoral parent may also lose his or her child's face. We often hear Chinese parents scold their children by asking where they expect their parents to show their (the parents') face. One important motivation for a child to excel in school is to enhance his or her parents' face. This mutual invocation of face also happens between students and teachers. The students with good academic performance enhance the teacher's face, and a teacher may also lose face over his or her students' poor performance.

Schoenhals points out that face is so central in Chinese social life that Chinese virtually make any performance a face arena and an evaluating ground. Performing well in school and on exams, particularly in the once-a-year college entrance exams, can entail enormous pressure for students and their families, especially for those with a good reputation to uphold and those from "intel-lectual" families.[25] During my clinic observation, I met several student patients whose illnesses were clearly related to feelings of loss of face or to the anxiety of potential loss of face involving exams and schoolwork. One young female patient was brought to the clinic by her mother who reported that after the daughter failed her college entrance exams, she suffered a mental trauma (*jing-shen ciji* 精神刺激), felt she could not show her face to the world anymore, and refused to come out of her room during the day. A patient who was a graduate student was worried so much about the coming English qualification exam that he developed a headache.

In the culture that makes *lian-mian* central to the concept of person, emo-tional expression itself is the performance of a person, which is subject to social evaluation and interpretation. What is important is not whether emotion is expressed or not, but in what context and how it is expressed. The relevant ques-tions are rather to whom, in what situation, with what purpose, and to what effect one expresses what emotions. As said above, those with higher status and higher expectations to live up to tend to be more sensitive to *mianzi* (social face) than those who do not have much *mianzi* in the first place. Those with high social status therefore tend to be more cautious about their behavior in public, including displaying their emotions. They tend to be more aware of the cultural norms regarding interpersonal behavior and cultural aesthetic values of connecting, appropriateness, and harmony. Demonstrating aggressiveness in public is considered low-status behavior. For a person with higher social status to engage him or herself in a public conflict is considered to "*diu mianzi* or *diu shenfen*" (lose face or social status). Therefore, a person with higher social status tends to disengage himself from those conflicts that get intense and ugly. However, those who do not have social status to lose usually tend to be more aggressive. Ironically, if through aggressiveness the lower status person is able to engage the higher status person in an argument at the same level, he actu-ally gains social face by dragging the other person down. So the higher status person who restrains from engaging in the conflict is said "not to give the other person face" (*bu gei lian* 不给脸). However, this does not mean that a person with higher social status will never display emotions inappropriately but rather that such display is subject to negative public sanction.

In any actual incidence, there may be several cultural factors at work involving social status, gender relations, and age difference. For example, when women grow older, they, at least among the less educated, become least restrained by face considerations and are expected to be more expressive and aggressive. When someone's face is threatened and attacked, he is expected to be angry. When a person loses a family member or a close friend, he is expected to demonstrate grief and sadness. In fact, when such demonstration is lacking, an explanation is called for. In the context of a village where the community is closely knit, sometimes the entire village is related in kinship terms, and everyday emotion experience may take different forms and styles. Emotional activities tend to be more observable. In addition, inappropriate display of emotions, at most, involves more of social face than moral face, and villagers care more about fulfilling their moral obligations toward each other than social prestige. They are more worried about a gift being returned or a favor being shared.

The communication of emotions in the clinical context is a slightly different matter. How a doctor and patient interact with each other depends on how they perceive the relationship. A senior doctor with a good reputation commands more trust from a patient than a younger doctor. In front of a doctor, a patient who normally occupies a lower status does not theoretically have much *mianzi* to lose. What makes the difference is if the doctor is perceived as "having a good attitude" (*taiduhao* 态度好), meaning being kind and understanding. Facing an understanding senior doctor, patients tend to express anger, sadness, and frustration quite freely. In fact, by the action of revealing his or her own emotions to the doctor and receiving emotional consoling, the impersonal doctor-patient relationship is somehow transformed into a more personal type of relationship. Once a woman in her thirties came to see the doctor at the clinic. They talked as if they were old friends. Then the doctor told her that the personal stamp she carved for him was of no use because she had the second character of his name carved incorrectly. He joked that after the many sessions that she had cried through, she did not even know the characters of his name. Their conversation was friendly and informal. Later, the doctor told me that this patient used to come to his office once a week. She was always the first to come to the clinic in the morning. As soon as she sat down, she started to cry. According to the doctor, she really cried, not just became teary-eyed, but cried loudly. She talked about her problems of infertility and family. She was depressed and suicidal. By the time I saw her, she had recovered and was back at work. In my field notes, I described her as "having a healthy facial complexion and talked and laughed at ease." She promised to carve a stamp for the doctor as a token of her gratitude. By revealing her emotions openly to the doctor, the young female patient presented herself not only as a patient that needed treatment for her illness but also as a suffering person who needed understanding and sympathy and thus defined and transformed this particular doctor-patient relationship.

Qing as Social Relations

A most commonly used emotion word is *ganqing* 感情. The term is composed of two characters: *gan* 感 (to feel, experience, or be moved) and *qing* 情 (feelings, emotions). The concept takes various meanings in Chinese everyday conversation, and its translation depends on the context in which it is used. What is unique about *ganqing* is its use is always embedded in specific dynamity of social relations as *qin qing* 亲情 (emotional attachment between family members), *fuqi qing* 夫妻情 (affection between husband and wife), *shisheng qing* 师生情 (feelings between teacher and student), *youqing* 友情 (friendship), and more. In this sense, *ganqing* is simply *renqing* 人情, which I translate as "human emotions existing in/as specific social relations." Hwang identifies *renqing* as the essential meaning of the Chinese concept of emotion,[26] and Kleinman and Kleinman clarify it as "a contextualized response, a response one feels in experiencing the concrete particularity of lived situations."[27] Yan suggests that *renqing* commonly has four different meanings. They are (1) human feelings which are basic emotional responses of an individual to everyday situations, (2) a set of social norms and moral obligations, (3) a favor, a gift, greetings, a visit and assistance, and (4) a social network. In short, *renqing* is seen fundamentally as social relations.[28]

Having a good relationship" in Chinese is actually "having good feelings" (*ganqing hao* 感情好) or simply "having feelings" (*you ganqing* 有感情). Though translated as "feelings," "to have *ganqing*" in this Chinese sense is not something simply "to have," but a process of "doing" a relationship in concrete social situations, and its communication therefore relies more on contextualized actions (*xing* 行) than merely on talk and speech (*yan* 言). The Potters notice that in Chinese culture, relationship is confirmed through the language of work and suffering rather than by referring to the emotion of love.[29] I can certainly see the point of the statement, but the problem with Potters' analysis is that it dichotomizes "work" and "affection" as if they are mutually exclusive in the Chinese experience. The result is a double reduction: "work" is stripped of its affective dimension, and "emotion," of its social significance. In fact, good feelings (*ganqing*) are best seen as unfolding through how one behaves within the social context. This is true especially among intimate relations. In these relations, *ganqing hao* is often described as *moqi* 默契 (tacit coordination between the parties developed through intimate interactions on a daily basis). Anticipating the other's needs and acting accordingly without being explicitly told is most valued as the true manifestation of *ganqing*. It takes a lot of good feelings to be aware of the situation that others are in and to care enough to take actions accordingly. It is in reciprocation of doing things for each other that *ganqing* is created and substantiated. "*Ganqing* exists only when sentiment, emotional attachment, and good feelings are felt by people involved in social interactions."[30] As Schoenhals points out, "[h]elping others to do things they cannot do alone, even mundane things, has great significance for the Chinese, as it is a primary means of expressing friendship and love."[31] Thus, the Chinese elderly like to receive gifts and help from their children and are proud of them because this not only lets them know that they are loved but also enhances the social face of the parents and the family. Refusing to reciprocate in sharing work is considered a "problem of emotions/feelings" (*ganqing wenti* 感情问题). One female informant complained that her husband never helped her with housework, not even when she was sick. She summarized the relationship as "lack of good feelings" (*mei ganqing* 没感情). For most Chinese, *ganqing* is expressed through actions taken and decisions made for each other on an everyday basis. A retired teacher described her relationship with one of her students as having good *ganqing*. After almost thirty years had passed, the student was still coming to visit her and brought her gifts on holidays.

When Chinese say that a person does not have *renqing* (human emotion) sensibility, they talk about a person's attitude and behavior toward others. A typical story involved a son who upon marriage took over his parents' apartment and forced the parents to make a bedroom out of the balcony. The story aroused emotional comments to the effect that the son was not a person, and he did not have a sense of *qinqing* (emotional attachment between family members), not to mention *renqing* in general. A positive example of having good *ganqing* involved a young couple who lived in the same building where I stayed while in Beijing. The neighbors would talk about them admiringly as "having really good relationship/feelings" (*ganqing zhenhao* 感情真好), comparable to saying that they really loved each other. They would mention such things as: every morning before he went to work, the husband would take the wife on the back of his bicycle to the bus stop, and in the evening he would wait at the bus stop and take his wife back home on his bicycle. What makes the community recognize this couple is the harmony and intimacy cultivated in mundane everyday experience. Good feelings, as recognized by family-oriented Chinese, come from familiarity and embody understanding that nurtures spontaneous coordination and cooperation among the members of a community.

Obviously, *renqing*, based on concrete social relations, is not conceptualized as something that can be isolated as "inner feelings." Chinese do have the concept of "*nei*" 内 (inside), yet *nei* exists meaningfully only when it is manifested to the outside. There is no meaningful inside that is without an outside correspondence in speech, action, or inaction. This inside and outside conceptualization is evident in the *zhongyi* mode of knowing, which is actually based on meticulous observations of the correspondence between functions of the inside *zang* 脏 (visceral systems) and the outside *xiang* 象 (outside manifestations). This inside is not understood as a fixed entity, but a process constantly in motion. In this sense, the outside manifestations can be seen as an integrative part of the same functional process. Interestingly, introspection (*neixing* 内省) in the

Chinese sense does not have the meaning of reaching deeply into oneself "for discovering the really real"[32] but refers to a morally oriented self-examination of one's behavior. A typical example of this type of self-examination comes from Zengzi, Confucius' disciple. He once said, "Everyday I examine (*xing* 省) myself on three counts: whether I have done my best working for others, whether I have kept my promise to friends, and whether I have appropriated and acted upon the teachings received from my teacher."[33]

Renqing is an interactional phenomenon, established, confirmed, and maintained through everyday reciprocation of favors, labor, care, food, assistance, kindness, and understanding. The relationship between parents and children is marked by the typical Chinese sense of mutual obligations and reciprocity. Chinese parents are known to put a major part of their resources and energy into their children's education and make great efforts to satisfy the children's needs. Children are expected to understand the parents' "labored heart" (*kuxin* 苦心) and appreciate their parents' efforts by being good students and honoring the parents' expectations. This is vividly captured in a newspaper article in which a ten-year-old girl told the reporter about her mother, whose job with a state-owned business had been cut:

> During the two years while my mother was out of work, she endured much hardship. In the afternoon and at night she worked in a restaurant. In the morning, she worked in another place. My relatives and friends all said that my mother seemed to become old suddenly. Not 40 yet, she has already lots of gray hair. I know my mother worked this hard for my sake. The way I can repay her is to study hard; otherwise I am not treating my mother right.[34]

The mother's response to the girl's words was that knowing the child cherished such a heart, all the hardship she suffered had been rewarded.

Qing as Social Norms and Moral Comments

The Chinese concept of emotion, captured in the expressions of *renqing* and *ganqing* is not something that is strictly opposite to reason (*li* 理) and moral significance (*yi* 义). The common expressions that Chinese use to advance their opinions, such as *juede* 觉得 or *gandao* 感到 have aspects of both thinking and feeling. Emotion, reason, and moral appropriateness are integrated in the Chinese language and experience. When a person is said not to understand human emotions (*butong renqing* 不通人情), the meaning may actually be that the person is not reasonable or does not act in accordance with common sense.

If we say that *renqing* is the human emotional response or sentiment embedded in a series of concrete social relations, then it can also be read as "a set of social norms and moral obligations" operative in everyday practices.[35] They are sometimes referred to as "affective reason" (*qingli* 情理) and "emotionally charged moral appropriateness" (*qingyi* 情义). Different social relations may evoke a different set of *li* (reasons) and *yi* (moral significance/appropriateness) that demand styles of behavior and of emotion appropriate to the relational context. Demonstrations of *qing* and the intensity of such demonstrations are justified or unjustified in the light of *li* and *yi,* which are contigent on the concrete social contexts. For example, a basic type of *qinqing* 亲情 (*ganqing* between family members) is *qing* between parents and children, which is traditionally characterized as *ci* 慈 (caring) for parents and *xiao* 孝 (filial piety) for children. In everyday life, *ci* and *xiao* are both emotions and codes of conduct.

In Chinese everyday language, idioms of emotions are frequently used in moral discourse. Anger is such an idiom. It is one of the frequently encountered emotions in the clinics of Chinese medicine. Many patients complain that their illness is "anger related" (*qide* 气的). If anger is considered a negative or stigmatized emotion that presents a potential threat to the existing social structure, why do people openly admit that they are angry to the extent of injuring their health? The Chinese tend to associate anger (*qi* 气, *nu* 怒) with illness and even death, as reflected in the Chinese saying that "one does not need to pay with his life if he 'angers' a person to death" (*qisiren bu changming* 气死人不偿命). This may seem to be an exaggeration, but Chinese often take it quite seriously. Many of them know the historical account of Zhu Geliang, the minister of the state of Shu who tricked Zhou Yu, the general of the state of Wu three times and finally "angered" him to death. Claiming to be angry is not to say that one feels personal frustration but to say that somebody else hurts a person by violating *qingli* or *qingyi.* A middle-aged female patient, a police officer, complained about her insomnia and the involuntary trembling of her hands. The trembling got worse when she was angry. After giving a description of her symptoms, she told the doctor that her illness resulted from anger caused by her mother-in-law (*bei popo qi de* 被婆婆气的), who, according to her, was not reasonable (*bu jiangli* 不讲理). According to her story, her mother-in-law's husband went to Taiwan just before 1949 and did not come back until recently. Now that the husband had returned, her mother-in-law became even more unbearable, as if the whole world owed her. Everybody in the family had to defer to her will, and she found fault with everybody, especially with her daughter-in-law. The patient commented that "it is true that my mother-in-law has suffered a lot from the political stigma and raising a child by herself, but that does not give her the right to make everybody else suffer." She also said that though she was very angry with her mother-in-law and really wanted to shout back at her to make her understand what she was doing, as a police officer (police officers and government officials are supposed to set good examples as civilized citizens), she could not do it. Others would say that if she could not handle her own family problem appropriately, how could she "take control of" (*guan* 管) others? By presenting herself as angry, she formulated her illness and emotion as a moral comment on her mother-in-law's violation of *qingli.* So by complaining that their illnesses are anger related, patients hold somebody else morally accountable for their sufferings—sufferings that are measurable in the "body."

Qing as Embodied Experience

Though the term *qingzhi* itself is used mostly in the context of Chinese medicine in reference to the function of emotions in relation to health and illness, the content of *qingzhi*, the so called "seven emotions" (*qiqing* 七情) or "five emotions" (*wuzhi* 五志) are concrete emotions that are part of everyday language and experience.[36] By glossing these emotions over as *qingzhi*, *zhongyi* doctors specify a medical context for talking about and evaluating emotions and finally transforming an experience of emotion into a treatable disorder.

Qingzhi, on the one hand, is unmistakably recognized as social in nature and always understood as the concrete emotions of *xi* 喜 (joy, happy), *nu* 怒 (anger, rage), *you* 忧 (sorrow, worries), *si* 思 (thinking, pensiveness), *bei* 悲 (grief), *kong* 恐 (fear), and *jing* 惊 (fright). These are "contextualized responses" of an individual "in experiencing the concrete particularity of lived situations."[37] Therefore, disordered *qingzhi*, though seen as having something to do with the patient's personal psycho-physiological dispositions (*bingfu* 秉赋) is often recognized by traditional Chinese medical doctors as closely and directly related to a person's social environment. My *zhongyi* teacher unequivocally marked interpersonal relationship (*renji guanxi* 人际关系) and inability to deal with it (*chuli bukai* 处理不开) as the main factors contributing to *qingzhi* disorders. He stressed that the ideal way to treat *qingzhi* disorders is to combine medical treatment (*yaowu zhiliao* 药物治疗) and persuasion (*quandao* 劝导) or disentanglement (*shuli* 疏理) of the patient's personal and emotional blockage in life. He believed that if he did not have to treat so many patients each day, he would be able to spend more time with each patient, and the efficacy would have been much better. Nowadays, this nonmedical method is also referred to as "psychological counseling" (*xinli zixun* 心理谘询). The more traditional method for such nonmedical treatment for *qingzhi* disorders is "treating an emotion with a counter emotion" (*yi qing sheng qing* 以情胜情). However, the so-called *xinli zixun* (psychological counseling) is different from the concept of psychological counseling in that it is not aimed at discovering and revealing intrapsychic conflicts, but it is more sociomorally oriented as fostering a "correct" or adaptive attitude and perspective in order for patients to handle their social situations better. Moreover, these "correct" insights into one's life are culturally embedded. Since Chinese medicine routinely incorporates nonmedical aspects into its clinical intervention, doctors, though spending limited time with their patients, seldom leave out the nonmedical part of *zhongyi* in their interaction with patients. This aspect will be discussed in detail in the following chapters.

Moreover, there is no doubt from the *zhongyi* point of view that *qingzhi* is embodied and experienced as dispersed *qi*, flares of liver, stagnated digestive functions, palpitations of the heart, and so on. Emotion and thought are seen as integrated parts of the human psycho-physiological process. As Sivin points out, Chinese do make a distinction between bodily and psychological functions when they feel it necessary, but Chinese physicians "were much more interested in their underlying integrity and interaction."[38] For them, changes in thought/feelings will have consequences in physiological changes, and therefore, experiential changes. The converse is also held to be true. Ots believes that there is a "correspondence of emotions and bodily complaints in psychosomatic disorders and suspects that through specific bodily symptoms or symptom patterns, *zhongyi* doctors may be able to identify some specific emotional changes.[39]

Without elaborated *zhongyi* language that connects emotive activities to specific bodily functional systems, ordinary Chinese talk about their emotions as the experience of *shenti* (body-person), which, as clear from the last chapter, is both body and person. It is very common for Chinese to calm their angry friends by saying, "Don't stay angry, or you will harm your *shenti*," or persuade somebody in grief to "restrain the feelings of grief" (*jieai* 节哀), or he will destroy his own *shenti*. Chinese believe that one's emotion is experienced in *shenti*, as they say "a smile makes you ten years younger, while worry brings you gray hair." The experience of a friend, an established middle-aged scholar, may illustrate how emotion/social/bodily changes are intertwined in real life experience. The following is translated from my notes of our conversation in the summer of 1994.

> For some time, I felt my *shenti* (body-person) was not good. I had insomnia, and I could not fall asleep at all. I was in low spirits (*qingxu buhao* 情绪不好) and was anxious and irritable all the time. I was afraid that my *shenti* might fall apart, and so I went to see *zhongyi* doctors. I was told that I had "nerves functional disorders" (*shenjing guannengzheng* 神经官能症). The doctor said my problem was related to "excessive worry and thinking" (*silu guodu* 思虑过度) that disturbed my spleen and stomach system (*piwei* 脾胃) and weakened my heart system and that I needed to take some Chinese herb medicine to modulate (*tiao* 调) my *shenti*. I thought he was right. During that period, Deng Xiaoping had just published his speech on his south inspection trips,[40] and the whole country was plunged into an economic frenzy. Everything became commercialized as if money was everything. I was constantly thinking about what I was going to do: follow the trend of "jumping into the sea of market economy" (*xiahai* 下海) like many others, or be content to be poor and do things I was good at? What would happen to an academic institution like ours that definitely could not survive the ups and downs of a market economy by itself? In those days I couldn't sleep well and had no desire for food. I was uncertain about the country's future and was worried about my future and my family's. This was the hardest period for me. I went to see *zhongyi* twice. The doctor prescribed some herbal medicine. After some time, I forget how long. . . . my symptoms mitigated. I am not sure if I was healed by the medicine or simply because I had thought things through and made my decision to stay within the academy.

The interconnections between feelings/thinking and bodily changes are meticulously coded in *zhongyi* physiology and considered essential in order to understand *qingzhi* disorders.

PHYSIOLOGY OF QINGZHI

As mentioned above, *qingzhi* refers specifically to seven emotions (*qiqing* 七情): happiness (*xi* 喜), anger (*nu* 怒), worry and anxiety (*you* 忧), thinking and obsession (*si* 思), sadness and grief (*bei* 悲), fear (*kong* 恐), and fright (*jing* 惊). In order to correspond to the functions of the five *zang* viscera, "seven emotions" are sometimes reduced to "five emotions" (*wuzhi* 五志) by consolidating *you* (worry) with *si* (obsession) and *kong* (fear) with *jing* (fright). Both 'qing' and 'zhi' can be translated as "emotions" and are frequently used in combination. However, some Chinese medical professionals recognize distinctions between *qing* and *zhi*.[41] They argue that *qing* are manifested emotions and *zhi* are latent. They are sometimes referred to as "internal emotion" (*neizhi* 内志) and "external emotion" (*waiqing* 外情). Yet, we should not mistake *zhi* as some sort of subconscious or hidden emotion. Rather *zhi* is understood as the "latent or neutralized" (*zhonghe* 中和) state in the process of emotions. In other words, 'qing' and 'zhi' are two terms referring to different stages of the same process.

Qingzhi and the Visceral Systems

Qingzhi is closely related to the functions of the visceral systems. *Neijing: Suwen* (The Inner Classics: Simple Questions) states that "a human being has five visceral systems which transform five kinds of *qi*; the five kinds of *qi* produce *xi* (joy), *nu* (anger), *bei* (sadness-grief), *you* (anxiety—sadness), and *kong* (fear)."[42] The seven emotions are also the external manifestations of the functions of the five visceral systems. Distinctions among the visceral systems influence changes in emotions, and emotional changes induce physiological changes. These emotional activities when kept in certain *du* (degree of intensity) are said to be normal phenomena. Only when activities of any of such emotions become excessive (*guoji* 过激) will emotion become pathological.

The visceral function systems in Chinese medicine fall into two categories: the five *yin* viscera (*wuzang* 五脏) and six *yang* viscera (*liufu* 六腑). The five *zang* viscera include the heart (*xin* 心), the lungs (*fei* 肺), the spleen (*pi* 脾), the liver (*gan* 肝), and the kidneys (*shen* 肾). Although designated as *yin* organs, they are the dominant functional systems in the holistic physiology of traditional Chinese medicine. The five *zang* systems are paired with six *fu* viscera: the small intestine (*xiaochang* 小肠), the large intestine (*dachang* 大肠), the stomach (*wei* 胃), the gallbladder (*dan* 胆), the urinary system (*pangguang* 膀胱) and the untranslatable *sanjiao* 三焦.[43] The *zang* and *fu* are considered as complementary in functions. It is characteristic of the physiological functions of the *zang* systems to transform (*shenghua* 生化) and store (*zhucang* 贮藏) vital essence and energy (*jingqi* 精气) and characteristic of the functions of the six *fu* viscera to accept, digest, transmit, and separate the water and food (*shuigu* 水谷). As shown in table 4.1, the five *zang* and the six *fu* systems join each other to form a complex of functions that links "all parts of the body in processes of producing normal and pathological effects."[44] *Zhongyi* physiology depends little on the knowledge of anatomy. *Zhongyi* theory of visceral systems is called "*zangxiangxue*" 脏象学 (studies of visceral system imagery) in which *zang* 脏 refers to the dynamic and relational processes of visceral systems of a living body and *xiang* 象 to be observable manifestations of the functions of the visceral processes. The Chinese medical theory stresses that the viscera in *zangxiangxue* are not anatomic concepts. "Most importantly they are the concepts that generalize the physiological and pathological functions of the bodily systems."[45] The phenomena that *zhongyi* investigates are different from those of biomedicine.[46] When a Chinese medical doctor is taking a pulse (*qiemai* 切脉), the attention is not on the pulse or the rhythmic dilating and contracting of arteries but on the movement of *mai*—the flow of *qi* and *xue* (blood) that sometimes resembles "a pearl rolling on a plate" and sometimes "water gushing out of a spring," registering the status of function and coordination of the visceral systems at the moment.[47]

The physiological correlations elaborated in *zangxiangxue* appear at several levels. First, each *zang* corresponds to a particular *fu* and interacts with other *zang* systems according to the *wuxing* sequence of influence to form a functional network of physiology. At another level, each *zang* system has its manifested configurations that are specifically related to certain sensual organs or surface openings to form continuity from the inside to the outside. For example, the tongue (*she* 舌) is called "the seedling of the heart." Changes in physiological functions of the heart system are said to manifest not only in color and coating of the tongue but also in taste and speaking.[48] We can still find another level of correlation. The physiological functions of the five *zang* systems are closely associated with human mental or "brain" activities including cognition and emotions. The heart is said to store *shén* 神 (spirit/consciousness) and is associated with the emotion of *xi* (joy, happiness); the liver system is said to store *xue* 血 (blood) and *hun* 魂 (ethereal soul) and is associated with the emotion of *nu* (anger, rage). Therefore, *zangxiangxue* of Chinese medicine not only specifies that the physiological functions of the five *zang* systems and the six *fu* systems are interconnected and that their equilibrium and harmony are essential for a healthy process of *shenti* but also indicates that the physiological network extends to include the mental and social environments through the demonstrated continuity from inside to outside and from *zangfu* systems to mental and emotional aspects of a person. Thus, the *zangxiang* system in fact implies a larger physiology of body-person that goes beyond the boundary of "physical body." This holistic physiology is the basic logic underlying *zhongyi*'s approach to *qingzhi* disorders.

Table 4.1 Summary of the Functions of the Five Visceral Systems

Zang *Visceral* System	*Affiliated* Fu System	*Governs & Unfolds in*	*Stores*	*Emotion Associated*	*Manifest & Vent*
Heart	Small intestine	Blood flow circulation tracks	*Shen* (spirit and vitality)	*Xi* (joy or happiness)	Manifests in face, vents at tongue
Spleen	Stomach	Transmission & transformation, flesh; muscles, four limbs	*Yi* (imagery)	*Si* (Worrying/thinking)	Manifests in lips, vents at mouth
Lung	Large intestine	Breathing	*Po* (sense; sensation)	*bei* (sadness/grief), *you* (anxiety/sadness)	Manifests in skin & body hair, vents at nose
Kidney	Urinary bladder & triple jiao	Fluids, marrow, bones	*zhi* (memory)	*kong* (fear), *jing* (startle, fright)	Manifests in hair, vents at ear, genitals, & anus
Liver	Gallbladder	Dredging & draining, dispersion upward and outward; sinews	blood *hun* (soul)	*nu* (anger)	Manifests in nails, vents at eyes

This table is based on information from Yet et. Al. 1983. Zhongyi Jichu

The physiology of the *zangfu* systems is systematized in terms of *wuxing* 五行 (the five transformative phases) into complicated cycles of production (*sheng* 生) and restraint (*ke* 克). Emotions, though viewed directly relevant to the heart system, are assigned separately to each one of the five visceral systems and are therefore subject to the same logic of interactions.

The Five Transformative Phases

Like *yin-yang* theory, "*wuxing*" is another ancient Chinese philosophical concept that has been integrated into the theoretical foundation of traditional Chinese medicine.[49] *Wuxing* are the characteristic activities of the five phases: wood, fire, earth, metal, and water. Because of the materialistic appearance of the five elements, it was routinely translated as the "five elements" and seen as comparable to the Greek four elements of earth, air, fire, and water, which are the ultimate roots of all natural things. However, as Sivin points out, *wuxing* are not elements in an "Aristotelian and medieval European form" but are "primarily concerned with process and change."[50] What links the five materials in nature to the five transformative phases is not what the five materials essentially are but what are observed to be characteristics of the former. Therefore, the wood phase of *wuxing* is characterized by the functions of growing (*shengzhang* 生长), dispersing upward and outward (*shengfa* 升发), and stretching and extending (*tiaoda shuchang* 调达舒畅). The fire phase is characterized by the functions of warming (*wenxu* 温煦) and rising (*shengteng* 升腾). The earth phase is characterized by the functions of transforming (*shenghua* 生化), carrying (*chengzai* 承载), and absorbing (*shouna* 收纳). The metal phase is noted for the functions of clearing (*qingjie* 清洁) and contracting (*shoulian* 收敛). Finally, the water phase is characterized as cooling (*hanliang* 寒凉), moisturizing (*zirun* 滋润), and moving smoothly downward (*runxia* 润下). All the effects that are perceived as characterized by the similar processes can be described with their respective phases. Thus the functions of the five-*zang* visceral organs are described in the language of *wuxing*.

Since the five phases are characteristically understood as processes and functions, what is important is not substance but relations: how each phase, in its own way, acts on other phases according to certain sequences. The forms of interactions are known as production (*sheng* 生), restraint (*ke* 克), violation (*hui* 侮) and encroachment (*cheng* 乘). Production means promotion of the function of the next phase in the sequence. The sequence of production of the five phases is the following: wood produces fire, fire produces earth, earth produces metal, and metal produces wood. In human physiological terms, the liver system facilitates the function of the heart system, the heart systems facilitates the spleen system, and so on. The sequence of restraint is the following: wood restrains earth, earth restrains water, water restrains fire, fire restrains metal, and metal restrains wood. Again, in physiological terms, the activities of the liver

Table 4.2   *Wuxing* and the Five-*Zang* Systems

Five Zang Systems	Wuxing	Characteristics
the Heart (*xin*)	Fire	Governing the flow of blood, having a warming function (*wenxuzhigong*).
the Spleen (*pi*)	Earth	Transforming the water & food (*yunhua shuiguo*), transfer refined nutrients (*shusong jingwei*), nourishing viscera and limbs and bones. Sources of generation of blood and *qi*.
the Lungs (*fei*)	Metal	Clearing and dredging (*shujiang*).
the Kidneys (*shen*)	Water	Moisturizing, cooling, moving downward, and constraining.
the Liver (*gan*)	Wood	Extending and reaching out (*xi tiaoda*), having function of spreading, and dredging (*shuxie gongneng*).

This table is based on Yin et al. 1983.

system restrain the activities of the spleen system, the spleen system restrains the kidney system, and so on.

Therefore, every single phase stands in four-way relations: producing and produced, restraining and restrained. For example, wood produces fire and is produced by water; it restrains earth but is restrained by metal. It is understood that through these interactions of generation and restraint the world obtains its harmony and balance. Yet Chinese are constantly aware that any of these activities may surpass its *du* (appropriate degree/intensity) and become excessive or may fall short in its *du* and become insufficient. This is when encroachment (*cheng*) and violation (*hui*) happen. For example, when the wood phase becomes too strong, it may exercise too much restraint on earth and weaken the function

Figure 4.1   The Sequence of Production and Restriction

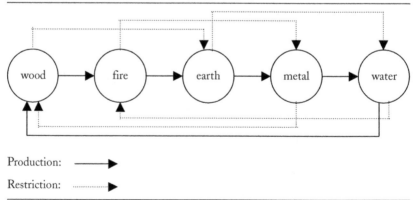

Production: ——▶

Restriction: ·········▶

This figure was originally used by Fred Blake in his lecture notes.

of the earth. This is known as encroachment. This may also happen when the activities of a phase are not sufficient and thus invite overrestraint. Violation happens when an overactive phase turns to suppress the function of the phase that is above it in the sequence of production. The result will be pathological imbalance. In this network of mutual influence, "a disorder appearing in one system can quickly ramify into others and produce symptoms implicating additional visceral systems or even masking the role of the visceral system that is its primary source."[51] In any given case, there are many possible positions for analyzing the pathological condition. The clinical action in this sense is always personal and contingent on the doctor's experience and strength.

However, *wuxing* reasoning together with *yin-yang* theory provides a unifying language and a practical guide for mapping the illness condition, anticipating the pathological development, and designing a therapy to effect a treatment. It certainly helped me to understand the *zhongyi* clinical language and to grasp the logic behind the doctors' clinical actions. I was impressed by Dr. Zhou's ability to tell the patients what symptoms they might have been experiencing and to get wholehearted confirmation from the patients. Once a surprised female patient asked Dr. Zhou how he could possibly know that she experienced lower abdominal pain and irregular menstruation before she told him, especially considering that he was a male doctor. Dr. Zhou laughed and said that knowledge came from his experience (*jingyan* 经验). He explained to me and his student doctors that an incompetent doctor sees a symptom as an isolated phenomenon, but no symptom appears in isolation. Since all the visceral systems are interconnected, certain symptoms always appear in correlation with others. For example, when the liver system is stagnant (*ganyu* 肝郁), a doctor should pay attention to the symptoms from the heart system. This is because, according to the *wuxing* model, the liver system as a wood phase facilitates the functions of the heart system, which is fire and will therefore possibly transmit the illness to the heart system. This is known as "the mother's sickness transmitted to the son" (*mu bing ji zi* 母病及子)."[52] So when the blood in the liver system is stagnant, it will fail to nurture (*ruyang* 濡养) the heart. Since the heart stores *shén* (spirit, manifested vitalities), when the heart *yin* is deficient, *shén* may lose its attachment (*shen shi suo gui* 神失所归), and the patient may experience insomnia, excessive dreams, or difficulty in concentration. Similarly, when the liver system is replete with fire (*ganhuo wang* 肝火旺), a doctor might need to think about the kidney system. It might be the deficiency of the kidney *yin* that results in excessive fire in the liver system. This is called "the water failing to immerse the wood" (*shui bu han mu* 水不涵木).[53] Dr. Zhou used a pot of boiling water as an example:

> When we hear the loud sound of the boiling water and see the enormous amount of steam coming out of the pot, we tend to think of the temperature as the only factor. But it is very likely that there is little water in the pot. In fact, less water will make a louder sound and more steam. What we do is to add

water. This is called "adding water to immerse the wood" (*zishui hanmu* 滋水 涵木). Clinically, this is to nourish the kidney *yin* to soften the liver system.

Wuxing reasoning has a particular role in treating emotional disorders. Since the emotions are said to be correspondent to specific functions of different visceral organ systems, they are also accountable in terms of the *wuxing* relationships. As shown in figure 4.3, sadness/grief is the emotion of the lungs, therefore, belonging to the phase of metal. Anger is the emotion of the liver, therefore, its mode is "metallic." According to the conquering or restraining sequence that metallic overcomes the wooden, the emotion of sadness/grief is said to overcome the emotion of anger. So when a person is excessively angry, bringing out the sadness may lessen the anger and thereby reduce the related symptoms. Such an emotional way of treating emotions is known as "treating emotions with emotions" (*yi qing sheng qing* 以情胜情), which can be found in the earliest medical records. According to *Neijing: Suwen* "anger hurts the liver, sadness overcomes it; . . . joy hurts the heart, fear overcomes it; . . . worry/thinking hurts the spleen, anger overcomes it; sadness hurts the lungs, joy overcomes it; fear hurts the kidneys, worry/thinking overcomes it."[54] Zhu Danxi (1281–58), a famous Yuan physician, was recognized for his skill at handling emotion-related disorders. One of Zhu's cases was retold by Zhang Jiebin (1560–1640), a renowned Ming physician, in his medical work, *Jingyue Quanshu: Yuzheng Mo* 景岳全书: 郁证谟 (*Complete Collection of Jingyue: Yu Illnesses*):

> After a girl was engaged, her fiancé went away on business. For two years, he had been away. Because of this, the girl did not eat and was lying in bed as if she was *chi* (of dementia). She had no other symptoms but lying in the bed facing the wall. This was due to the fact that her persistent longing and thinking (*si*) caused *qi* to congeal (*jie*). Medicine could not be effective by itself. [The doctor reasoned] that when there was joy (*xi*), the illness could be remitted, or she could be made angry so that the *qi* of wood could rise and extend and the *qi* of spleen would open. This was because wood could restrain earth. Therefore, the physician went to the girl and provoked her into rage. She cried for quite a long time and was given a bag of herbal medicine. After that, the girl asked for food. Though her illness was remitted, only joy could cure her completely. Therefore, an arrangement was made for her fiancé to return. After that, the illness did not recur.

Zhang Congzheng (1156–1228), a physician of the Yuan, was also known to be good at using emotions to treat emotions (see table 4.3).[55] The following are two cases from his book *Rumen Shiqin* 儒门事亲 (The Confucian Way of Caring for One's Parents, compiled during 1217–21):

> Guan's wife had a strange illness. She did not eat and had a bad temper. She was often heard shouting angrily. Many doctors were invited but failed to cure her. Zhang was invited. After an examination, he told the husband that his wife's illness could not be cured only by medicine, but had to use the

Table 4.3 Emotions and Counteremotions

Emotions	Transformative Phase	Correspondent Visceral System	Emotion That Overcomes
Anger (nu)	Wood	Liver	Worry
Anxiety/thinking (si)	Earth	Spleen	Fear
Fear/fright (kong/jing)	Water	Kidney	Joy
Joy (xi)	Fire	Heart	Sadness/grief
Sadness/grief (you/bei)	Metal	Lung	Anger

methods of "curing emotion with an emotion." Then two actor/dancers were invited. They put on makeup and performed in front of the wife. The patient was induced to laugh. The second day, these two actors put on makeup and performed wrestling. This made the patient laugh unceasingly. At the same time, the doctor had two women with good appetites sitting beside the wife. While eating joyfully, they complimented each course of food. By this, the patient began to want food. After a few days, her appetite improved, and her anger was cured too.

Another case involved a wife from a rich family who suffered insomnia for three years. No medicine was effective.

Doctor Zhang Congzheng was invited. He diagnosed that the illness was the result of excessive worrying and thinking due to the task of taking care of a large extended family. He decided that the illness could only be cured by emotion. He arranged a cure with the husband. The doctor accepted a lot of money from the husband and in front of the wife, lived and feasted in the house for days, and left without leaving a single prescription. The wife was outraged and then began sweating. That very night she fell into a deep sleep and did not get up for eight to nine days. After that, the wife was cured. This is the case of "anger overcomes worry."

This ancient method of emotion being cured by counteremotion can still be found in contemporary zhongyi practice. An author of a popularized zhongyi book tells the story of his own experience in treating a pregnant female patient. The patient came to seek help for her obsession with a past experience. She was troubled by the image of her high school male teacher who had hugged her in an inappropriate way. The image of this teacher refused to go away. Drawing on theories that xi (usually translated as "joy," but here is better translated as "excitement") that injures the heart can be overcome by fear and mitigated by anger, the author (the doctor) began by accusing the teacher of having made an unforgivable mistake and being irresponsible. Doing this, he managed to make the woman angry at the teacher. Then he started to point out that she had a loving husband and was expecting a baby and asked her to think about the consequence for her coming baby and her family if she indulged herself in unrealistic fantasy. By resorting to the emotion of anger and fear, the author successfully helped the patient to let go of the past.[56]

Qingzhi and Transformative *Qi*

What is really transformative in *zhongyi* physiology is *qi* which is translated variously as "air," "breath," and "vital energy". *Qi* is defined in contemporary *zhongyi* textbooks as "the material basis of life." Since *qi* itself is constantly in motion and in transformation, and it promotes (*tuidong* 推动) the activities of life and functions to warm up (*wenxu*) the body, *zhongyi* explains human physiological changes and activities in reference to the changes and transformations of *qi*.[57] Although *qi* is defined as "material," yet it is not a tangible or measurable entity. What is central about *qi* is what it does—its functions. They are summarized as promoting (*tuidong*) human physiological activities, keeping up (*wenxu*) the body's temperature, defending (*fangyu* 防御) the body from the invasion of "heteropathic *qi*" (*xieqi* 邪气), reinforcing and conserving (*gushe* 固摄) the vital substance of the body, and transforming (*qihua* 气化) bodily substances.[58] Normal functions are achieved through orderly motions of *qi* characterized as moving up, going down, coming in, and going out. The dynamic balance is upset if the certain *qi* is supposed to go up but goes down instead, or if certain *qi* moves too fast or too slow. For example, the heart *qi* goes down, while the kidney *qi* is going up. The liver *qi* spreads out while the lung *qi* clears downward. When the movement of *qi* is obstructed, the result is the disordered *qi* mechanism, such as stagnation, congestion, blockage, and closure of *qi*, which lead to all kinds of somatic and psychological symptoms.

Qingzhi functions are also understood in terms of *qi* transformations. The emotional impact on bodily processes is not significant in terms of chemical changes but in terms of altered *qi* movement. For example, when angry, *qi* moves up; when happy, *qi* is relaxed; when sad, *qi* is dissipated; when scared, *qi* moves down; when startled, *qi* is disturbed; and when thinking too hard, *qi* tends to congeal. Excessive emotional activities are said to upset the normal motion of *qi* relevant to its specific visceral functions. Once excessive emotions are sustained for long, the circulation of *qi* is obstructed, and the functions of visceral systems are disturbed, which results in various physical and psychological symptoms. With excessive emotions as clear illness factors, the disorders are very likely described as *qingzhi bing* (emotion-related disorders). However, the *zhongyi* clinical process understood as "differentiating patterns and determining treatment" (*bianzheng lunzhi* 辨证论治) should not be confused with the diagnostic process found in biomedical settings as labeling the disease and matching it with a standardized treatment. The following chapters focus on the *zhongyi* clinical process of *bianzheng lunzhi* and discuss how a particular diagnosis is arrived at and a treatment is determined.

V

Understanding *Zhongyi* Clinical Classification

When I first started my fieldwork at the hospital, I was confident that through my participant observation in the actual clinic settings, the picture of *qingzhi bing* 情志病 (emotion-related disorders) would present itself clearly to me and that it would not be difficult for me to define and classify various *qingzhi* disorders according to how they are organized in actual clinical settings. I remember that I was anxiously waiting for the doctor to give a diagnosis after he examined the patients. I was concerned about how a group of symptoms were associated with a particular illness and if this particular illness was considered a *qingzhi* disorder. To my great disappointment, despite my diligent notetaking, these two categories of information remained mostly blank in my notes. I noticed that diagnosis in terms of labeling an illness was not a necessary part of *zhongyi* clinical process at all, and it did not make a significant difference in determining therapy if a given illness was a *qingzhi* disorder or not. Several times, I directly asked the doctor exactly what illness he was diagnosing or treating. This was apparently a layperson's (*waihang* 外行) question, for the doctor would answer my question as he did those patients who pressed for an illness name. He would say that according to Western medicine, it was neurosis (*shenjing guanneng zheng* 神经官能症, literally, "nerves functional disorder") or "vegetation nerves out of balance" (*zhiwushenjing shitiao* 植物神经紊乱). Answers to my question of whether a case belonged to the category of *qingzhi bing* were usually ambiguous. Frequently, I was told that a certain case was related to *qingzhi*.

Not until sometime into my clinical observation did I begin to realize that the whole time I was trying to read the *zhongyi* clinical process in terms of the "biomedical way of thinking" (*xiyi siwei fangshi* 西医思维方式)," which my *zhongyi* teacher had cautioned against at the very beginning of my clinical observation. I automatically assumed that *zhongyi* clinical work would lead to the diagnosis of an illness based on the presence or absence of certain distinctive symptoms and the matching of the illness with an herbal prescription. Apparently, *zhongyi* diagnosis does not always involve creating a clear-cut taxonomy by appealing to a few distinctive features that mark phenomena belonging to the same category. The classificatory logic of the *zhongyi* clinical process that transforms the disordered *qingzhi* into an ordered pattern of an illness needs to be understood in light of a different mode or tradition of knowing. The focus of this tradition has been preeminently eventful or processual as discussed in the previous chapters. It is not that *zhongyi* clinicians are not able to understand the world structurally, but rather that their priority has been given to movements (*dong* 动) and changes (*bianhua* 变化). Scientific rigor and structural intelligibility have to give way to the readiness of accounting for dynamic relations and situational concreteness.

The central part of *zhongyi* clinical work is summarized as *bianzheng lunzhi* 辨证论治 (pattern differentiation and therapy determination) or *bianzheng shizhi* 辨证施治 (pattern differentiation and therapy application) in contemporary *zhongyi* writings. *Bianzheng* is to differentiate patterns of syndromes and therefore is a form of *zhongyi* classificatory technique. Determination of an effective therapeutic action (*lunzhi*) depends on accurate *bianzheng*. A textbook starts with:

> One distinctive feature of *zhongyi* clinical process of treating illnesses is *bianzheng lunzhi*. The practice of so-called "treating same illness with different therapies" (*tong bing yi zhi* 同病异治) and "treating different illnesses with the same therapies" (*yi bing tong zhi* 异病同治) takes *zheng* 证 (patterns/ syndromes) as its basis. Therapies change when *zheng* changes.... The focus is all on *zheng*, also known as *zhenghou*.[1]

The Chinese medical concept of "*zheng*" is not the same as the biomedical concept of "syndrome". Similarly, *bing* is not the *zhongyi* equivalent of disease. To understand the pivotal process of *bianzheng luzhi*, we need to understand a set of related concepts: "*zheng*" 症 (symptoms/signs), "*zheng*" 证 or "*zhenghou*" 证候 (patterns),[2] and "*bing*" 病 (illness/disorder). Judith Farquhar's *Knowing Practice* (1994) offers a detailed and systematic analysis of the clinical process of syndrome/pattern differentiation and therapy determination. Her analysis of the temporal form of *kanbing* 看病 (looking at the illness) is particularly relevant to my description of *zhongyi* classification. In the following passages, especially in those discussing symptom and syndrome differentiation, her work is frequently referenced. Scheid's recent book has one chapter on *bianzheng lunzhi*, which offers a detailed account of the modern evolution of the concept and is also an important source of reference for the analysis in this chapter.[3]

ZHENG (SYMPTOMS), ZHENG (PATTERNS), AND BING (ILLNESSES/DISORDERS)

In contemporary *zhongyi* texts, *zheng* (symptom), *zheng* (pattern), and *bing* (illness/disorder) are discussed as three different but related medical concepts. They all reflect pathological conditions resulting from "loss of yin-yang balance of lived body" (*renti zishen de yinyang pingheng* 人体自身的阴阳平衡)

and "disturbed equilibrium between internal and external environments" (*nei-wai huanjing tongyi xing zhang'ai* 内外环境统一性障碍) but have differential significance in relation to the clinical process of diagnosis.[4]

The term *zheng* (symptom) refers to various anomalies (*yizhang ganjue* 异常感觉) experienced by the patient and external manifestations (*waibu biaoxian* 外部表现) of pathological changes observed by the doctor. They provide the basis for the doctor to differentiate patterns and diagnose illnesses.[5] Farquhar makes a further distinction between *zheng* 征 (signs) and *zheng* (symptoms). Not following the conventional biomedical distinction between "objective signs" and "subjective symptoms," Farquhar's separation of *zheng* (signs) from *zheng* (symptoms) is rather temporal. *Zheng* 征 are signs initially reported and presented to the doctor by the patient or directly elicited from the patient by the doctor. The signs of illness are then processed by the doctor and turned into "medicalized" *zheng* (symptoms), which bear conventional medical implications. In a biomedical setting, the distinction might be more significant since some of the signs may not be taken as relevant symptoms of a particular disease. In a *zhongyi* clinic, what the patient reports and what the doctor takes as symptoms are not significantly different, and the temporal transition from signs to symptoms is usually unmarked. *Zhongyi* physicians do not categorically separate (sign) from the symptom, but rather use *zheng* (symptom) to mean both signs and symptoms. Symptoms recognized in a *zhongyi* clinic, such as "palpitation" (*xinhuang* 心慌), "shortness of breath" (*qiduan* 气短), or "restlessness" (*zuowo bu an* 坐卧不安), are very much descriptive and experiential, and the patient's voice remains authoritative regarding what are medically significant symptoms. Farquhar also recognizes that the patient's own narrative of his illness "plays a major role in delimiting the nature of the illness for both doctor and patient."[6] In *zhongyi* clinics, a patient is invited to report on whatever signs and symptoms she or he experiences. Any reported symptom is accepted as legitimate and contributing to the understanding of the whole pathological condition. This contrasts sharply with the clinical process in a biomedical hospital, where since a disease is understood as a discrete entity with clear boundaries, only certain signs and symptoms are accepted as legitimate or relevant.

An incident that happened to one of my friends brought me to this awareness. He had an acute migraine and was introduced to a doctor working at a prestigious biomedical hospital in Beijing. Afterward when I talked to the doctor, the doctor asked if my friend was really a college professor and said that he behaved like an old peasant who did not know how to *kanbing* (look at illness). My friend complained about a headache and then moved on to talk about his back pain and then jumped to complain about his stomach and later mentioned his vexation and irritability and his sweaty hands and feet. The doctor had to remind him what he was there for. In a disease-oriented biomedical clinic, sweaty hands and feet are perceived as bearing little relevance to a of migraine. However, in *zhongyi* clinics, such patient behavior is perfectly normal and expected. Not just common complaints, but idiosyncratic complaints are also treated with the same seriousness. Once I was amused by a patient who complained that he could feel his heart beat everywhere on his body, and he insisted that wherever on his body he touched, he could count his heartbeat. Afterward, the doctor seriously said to me that we healthy people may never experience what a patient experiences, but that does not mean what the patient experiences is not real or relevant.

Zheng (symptoms) are subject to further abstraction and generalization and are made "amenable to perception as a pattern."[7] This pattern is then called "*zheng*" (证). The step from *zheng* (symptoms) to *zheng* (pattern/syndrome) is referred to as "*bianzheng*" (pattern differentiation). This *zheng* is also called "*zhenghou*" 证候, where the second character implies a configuration of various factors observed over a period of time. The same character is used in the term *qihou* 气候 (climate). Based on the pattern of the syndrome, a therapeutic method is determined, which is known as *lunzhi* (therapy determination). Together, this process is referred to as "*bianzheng lunzhi*" or simply "*zhengzhi*" 证治 (syndrome differentiation and therapy determination). Different from symptoms and illnesses, *zheng*, as syndrome configurations, refers more to "patterns of history" that "characterize a group of symptoms typical of a particular condition or disturbance" than to the "structure of the body or disease."[8]

The classificatory principles of the clinical process of *bianzheng* (differentiation of patterns) summarized in contemporary *zhongyi* textbooks include "the eight rubrics differentiation" (*bagang bianzheng* 八纲辨证), "the visceral system functions differentiation" (*zangfu bianzheng* 脏腑辨证), "illness factors differentiation" (*bingyin bianzheng* 病因辨证), "six types differentiation" (*liujing bianzheng* 六经辨证),[9] and "defensive, active, constructive, and blood *qi* differentiation" (*wei, qi, ying, xue bianzheng* 卫气营血辨证). Of all these aspects for consideration, the eight rubrics are basic differentiation guidelines known as determining "the core syndrome patterns" (*hexin zhenghou* 核心症候).[10] The eight rubrics consist of four pairs of polaric relations: *yin* and *yang*, exterior (*biao* 表) and interior (*li* 里), cold (*han* 寒) and hot (*re* 热), and depleted (*xu* 虚) and replete (*shi* 实). This system of pattern differentiation is said to reflect the quality or nature of an illness (*bing xing* 病性). Liu Yanchi summarizes the eight guiding principles of differentiation as

- *yin* and *yang*, which describe the general type of the illness.

- interior and exterior, which describe the location of the illness.[11]

- cold and heat, which describe the specific nature of the illness.

- deficiency and excess, which describe the state of the struggle between anti-pathogenic *qi* and the pathogenic factor.[12]

These guidelines provide the preliminary dimensions for organizing symptoms. Yet not only do these differentiation methods allow many different combinations, but also the qualities of *yin* and *yang* constantly shift so that the exterior may move inward and the interior outward, and repletion may turn into depletion. In addition, from either end of a polaric pair, there is continuity and difference in degree. Therefore, any syndrome differentiation according to the eight guidelines is a description of an illness condition in time. The actual clinical differentiation of syndromes is always flexible. As is generally recognized by *zhongyi* doctors, "the principle of suiting the measures to the specific conditions of the person, the illness, the time and space, . . . is not only clinically necessary, but is also where the quintessence of *zhongyi*'s way of thinking lies."[13]

In addition to the eight rubrics as basic diagnostic methods for the differentiation of syndromes, the states of *qi* and *xue* (blood) are also most frequently considered dimensions in the process of pattern differentiation. Together with the eight principles, they are considered as reflecting the quality and nature of an illness process. For *qi*, the considerations are on its movement: deficient (*xu* 虚), sinking (*xian* 陷), stagnation (*zhi* 滞), or adverse (*ni* 逆), and so on. For blood, similarly, the qualities of its flow and functions are considered, such as deficiency, stagnancy, and congestion.

A group of symptoms can also be subject to further differentiation according to the dimensions of the visceral functions. This process of differentiation is said to describe the illness location (*bingwei* 病位). A basic name for any syndrome differentiation at least includes two types of information, that is, the nature and the location of a disorder.[14] For example, the syndrome of liver stagnation (*ganyu* 肝郁) uses two characters to describe the nature of the disorder, which is the stagnant flow of *qi* and the affected visceral system, the liver.[15] Other aspects are also involved in the process of differentiation of patterns, such as illness-factor differentiation (*bingyin bianzheng*), which includes the factors of the six excesses (*liu yin* 六淫): wind, cold, heat, dampness, dryness, and fire, and the seven emotions (*qiqing* 七情). There are always more aspects to look at as is necessary in the real clinical situation. As we discern more dimensions for consideration, it becomes more difficult to construct an unambiguous taxonomical hierarchy. In fact, the different methods of *zhenghou* differentiation should not be understood as taxonomic. They are best understood as practical and pedagogical guidelines for clinical actions, as Farquhar argues.[16] They offer various dimensions for clinicians to think about and to refer to when mapping out the underlying conditions of physiological and pathological changes and when designing therapeutic principles and formula.

There are endless possibilities in terms of clinical manifestations and the direction of an illness's development over time. The doctor's understanding of the nature of a particular pattern and its possible transformation, and the methods of intervention available to deploy, rely heavily on an individual doctor's knowledge, experience with similar symptom configurations, and flexibility and creativity.

As Farquhar points out, the *zhongyi* clinical work

> entails a great attentiveness to temporality, an understanding of illness developments and healing techniques as process. This stands in contrast to a

medicine of anatomical structures and fixed lesions, reductive causality, and mechanical influence.... A focus on the clinical work of Chinese medicine that privileges the practical and the temporal reveals Chinese medical classification as a method of deploying material from the medical archive within specific projects of healing, a continuing subordination of formalized knowledge to the concrete demands of the moment.[17]

The attentiveness to temporality and processual nature of differentiation of syndrome patterns also characterizes *zhongyi* classificatory logic and methods. In view of the language of *yinyang* and the five transformative phases that characterize the dynamic network of Chinese psychophysiology and pathology, any classificatory statement is a temporal and spatial description of dynamic configurations of the manifestations of an illness condition. Such configurations captured at one time are subject to constant reconfigurations. Thus one *zheng* may shift to another.[18]

Zhenghou thus conceptualized poses a fundamental difficulty for standardization of pattern differentiations based on the modern scientific classificatory systems that underlie the biomedical diagnosis of disease. In the last two decades, *zhongyi* scholars have shown increased concerns as to how to make classification of *zhenghou* more scientifically rigorous and at the same time to retain its characteristics of flexibility, concreteness, and pragmaticity.[19] By the standards of modern scientific nosological principles, the present practices require considerable improvement. In fact, continuous attempts have been made to standardize the concepts and classification of *zhenghou*.[20] Yet it is also realized that if *zhongyi* adopts modern nosological principles to bring differentiation of patterns of syndromes closer to modern scientific classification as has been pushed and experimented recently, these highly systematic and standardized categories and types, though more accessible to students in modern classroom learning, will then be more arbitrary (*renwei xing* 人为性), will be less reflective of the complexity of actual interrelatedness and transformations among symptoms and syndrome patterns, and most of all, will detach the classification from the concrete clinical work that takes practice as its guide.[21]

Many contemporary debates of *bianzheng* involve distinctions and relations between *zheng* (patterns/syndromes) and *bing* (illness/disorder). *Bing* is also called "*jibing*" 疾病, which is more formal.[22] Roughly, there have been about four thousand illness names recognized in *zhongyi*.[23] Some of these illness names still have value and are used in today's *zhongyi* clinics. In fact, a typical textbook of *zhongyi* internal medicine (*neike* 内科) is organized according to illness names.[24] However, *zhongyi* illness names are not clearly defined categories based on a set of consistent criteria and systematic methods. *Bing* (illness/disorder), *zheng* (symptoms), and *zheng* (pattern/syndromes) in many cases are not mutually exclusive categories. For example, cough (*kesou* 咳嗽) and palpitation (*xinji* 心悸) are referred to as "*bing*" in *zhongyi* textbooks, but they are not completely different from symptoms. Sometimes illness names are used to indicate patterns and syndromes. For example, the six cold damage illnesses (*shanghan liujing bing* 伤寒六经病) are talked about as *bing*, but many scholars and physicians see them as *zheng* (patterns) reminiscent of the eight rubrics.[25] At other times, the names of *zheng* (patterns) are used to designate *bing* (illnesses), such as block of dampness (*shizu* 湿阻) and liver *qi* stagnation (*ganyu* 肝郁). Occasionally, one illness name corresponds to only one pattern, and "differentiation of illness" then equals "differentiation of patterns."[26] According to Chen Xiaoye, the distinction between *zheng* and *bing* is relative, and they are not categorically different concepts. When a condition is talked about as "an object of investigation" (*renshi duixiang* 认识对象), it is habitually referred to as "*bing*," but as "the result of investigation" (认识结果), it is more likely to be referred to as "*zheng*."[27] The difference is rather positional than conceptual.

A pathological condition may be described as *bing* or *zheng*, but when coming to determination of treatment (*lunzhi* 论治) and designing drug formulas (*nifang yong yao* 拟方用药), it is the differentiation of *ben* 本 (the root) of the disorder experienced by the particular patient that matters most.[28] This *ben* as "the result of a medical investigation" captures the temporal and concrete pathological changes manifested in a particular patient and at a particular stage and is very often presented in the language of "yin-yang imbalance" (*yin-yang shitiao* 阴阳失调), "the relative advances and retreats between the body's own orthopathic and heteropathic forces" (*zheng-xie xiaozhang* 正邪消长), and "patterns of bodily functional changes" (*jineng bianhua tedian* 机能变化特点). In this sense, the *ben* of a disorder corresponds largely to contemporary *zhongyi* articulation of *zheng* (patterns).[29] Chen Xiaoye, in his article on the uniformity of *zheng* (pattern) and *bing* (illness), also argues that there have not been two separate systems of *bianzheng* (differentiation of patterns) versus *bianbing* (differentiation of illnesses) in *zhongyi* diagnostics.[30] Diagnosis in terms of illness names in *zhongyi* then is not as significant as in biomedicine. It bears little relevance in determining a specific treatment. As long as the doctor can reach an accurate *bianzheng* (pattern differentiation), a therapeutic strategy can be determined and a remedy can be found.[31] Very often, illness names are left out of the doctor's written records, which routinely include key symptoms, differentiation of syndrome patterns, therapeutic principles, and herb prescriptions.

REDEFINING *BIANZHENG LUNZHI*

Nothing is superficial about *zhongyi*'s claim that *bianzheng lunzhi* (differentiating patterns and determining therapies) is a defining feature of *zhongyi* clinical practice and that *bian zheng* is fundamentally different from *bian bing* 辩病 when *bing* is defined in the biomedical sense of disease. Contemporary *zhongyi* scholars trace the theorized practice of *bianzheng lunzhi* to *Shanghan Zabing Lun* 伤寒杂病论 (Discussions of Cold Damage and Various Disorders) by the East Han scholar-physician Zhang Zhongjing (150–219 AD). This classic treatise is said to have established the principle of *bianzheng lunzhi*. The procedure of differentiating patterns and determining specific herbal formulas based on "*liu-jing*" 六经 (the six types)[32] contains core elements similar to "*ba gang bianzheng*" (the eight rubrics differentiation) outlined in contemporary *zhongyi* texts.[33] However, the use of the terms of *bing* (illnesses) and *zheng* (patterns) was not systematically defined. Disorders were grouped and named generally as *bing*, and formulas were usually designated as *zheng*–specific patterns of disorders (*yi fang ming zheng* 以方名证). The late Ming scholar-physician Zhang Jiebin (1560–1639) is another historical figure credited with major contributions to the development of the *bianzheng lunzhi* principle. His pattern differentiation theory based on "*liang gang*" 两纲 (two rubrics of yin-yang) and "*liubian*" 六变 (six variations of internal and external, depletion and repletion, and cold and hot) led to "*bagang bianzheng*" (pattern differentiation based on the eight rubrics), one of the major methods of pattern differentiation used today.[34] Other forms of differentiating patterns were also practiced and theorized in the history of Chinese medicine. Zhang Yuansu (1151–1234), the scholar-physician of Jin, is credited with establishing the theory of "*zangfu bianzheng*" (pattern differentiation based on the visceral systems). The Qing scholar-physician Ye Tianshi (1667–1746) is recognized for developing the theory of "*wei, qi, ying, xue bianzheng*" (differentiation based on defensive, active, constructive, and blood *qi*).[35]

It seemed that generations of Chinese scholar-physicians used '*bing*' (illness) and '*zheng*' (pattern) flexibly in an unexamined manner and concerned themselves more with how to capture the temporal and spatial changes of a pathological process for the purpose of determining an effective therapy. Indeed, before the Western "anatomoclinical medicine" was introduced and spread in China in the early twentieth century, there seemed to be no compelling need to systematically distinguish *zheng* (patterns) and *bing* (illnesses) and no apparent reasons for Chinese scholar-physicians to reflect on distinctive features of their own profession. For them, tracing the problem to its sources (*qiu ben* 求本) through differentiating *yin-yang*, interior and exterior, depletion and repletion, and environmental and other factors constituted "the natural way of doing medicine" (yidao 医道). Only when it was challenged by the unfamiliar and powerful knowledge system of "the medical other" did *zhongyi* practitioners began to "discover" what was distinctive about the theory and practice of their own profession, and the distinctive meanings of Chinese medical concepts, including the diagnostics of *bianzheng*, were then made available to consciousness.

Similarities and differences between *zhongyi* and *xiyi* became commonly debated issues in the 1920s and 30s in medical circles, such as, *zhongyi* differentiates patterns (*zhongyi bian zheng* 中医辨证), and Western medicine differentiates diseases (*xiyi bian bing* 西医辨病). Zhang Xichun (1860–1933), the earliest advocate for "integrating Chinese and Western medicine," stated "the way western medicine uses drugs is to seek localized effect and the emphasis is on symptoms of an illness [*bing zhi biao* 病之标]; the way Chinese medicine uses drugs is to seek the causes and the emphasis is on the roots of an illness [*bing zhi ben* 病之本]. Yun Tiejiao (1878–1935), another early advocate for integrating Chinese and Western medicine, also pointed out that the physiology of Western medicine is based on anatomy (*xiyi zhi shengli yi jiepou* 西医之生理以解剖), and the physiology of Chinese medicine originated from the Inner Classics is based on transformation of *qi* (*"Neijing" zhi shengli yi qihua* 内经之生理以气化).[36] Against this historical background, *bianzheng lunzhi* (differentiation of patterns and determination of therapies) began to emerge as the diagnostic principle that centrally reflects Chinese medical theory (*yi li* 医理) and defines its practice.

However, it was not until 1958, in the first national textbook, *Zhongyixue Gailun* 中医学概论 (Outline of Chinese Medicine), that *bianzheng lunzhi* as the defining feature of *zhongyi* was first clearly stated. The reconstruction of *bianzheng lunzhi* was made possible by the fundamental transformation in the *zhongyi* profession in the 1950s. This included reorganization of space of *zhongyi* practice into modern hospitals, a newly defined status of *zhongyi* as comparable to biomedicine in the public health systems, the established relationship between the *zhongyi* institution and the state, and the newly acquired vocabulary of "dialectics" (*bianzhengfa* 辩证法) to articulate *zhongyi* theories and methods.[37] Scheid argues that *bianzheng lunzhi* became important because it accomplished several goals: allowing *zhongyi* professionals to define their profession as categorically different from Western medicine and thus promising a possible solution for the integration of two medicines; establishing a connection with the cultural tradition that is politically appropriate; and facilitating the systematic teaching of Chinese medicine in the newly institutionalized *zhongyi* education.[38] For many veteran scholar-physicians, who had been instrumental to redefining *zhongyi* before and after the 1950s, the concept of *bianzheng lunzhi* quintessentially embodies *zhongyi siwei fangshi* 思维方式 (way of thinking). From this way of thinking, illness is approached as an event of loss of equilibrium resulting from dynamic interactions between a person's own positive/defensive ability (*zheng* 正) and pathogenic forces (*xie* 邪), and treating illnesses entails using whatever way to alter the dynamics and to facilitate positive changes leading to gaining a new balance, that is, health.

ZHONGYI ILLNESS NAMES AND QINGZHI DISORDERS

The *zhongyi* illness categorization is still considered valuable in diagnostics, despite several efforts to abolish the *zhongyi* illness nosology and to adopt the more scientific disease classifications of biomedicine. Then, in what way is a *zhongyi* illness name functional and meaningful? It should be clear that a *zhongyi* illness name is not used in the same way as a is diagnosis in a biomedical setting, where a diagnosed disease is generally matched with a prescription of therapy with little consideration for an individual patient's psycho-physical and social particularities. However, *zhongyi lunzhi* (determination of therapy)

relies predominantly on differentiation of these particularities. According to
the contemporary *zhongyi* textbooks, illnesses (*bing*) and patterns (*zheng*) are
practically related. A correctly diagnosed illness name can help the doctor to
gain an overall understanding of changes of an entire pathological process and
to determine a general therapeutic strategy. For instance, if a pathological condition is classified as "phlem-rheum illness" (*tanyin bing* 痰饮病), a physician
then knows that since all patterns of phlem-rheum illness are caused by "*yin*
pathogenic factors" (*yin xie* 阴邪) and are cold (*han* 寒) in nature, the general
therapeutic strategy should be "using warm drugs to harmonize it" (*yi wenyao
he zhi* 以温药和之). Yet whether to use a warm drug or not or what warm drugs
to use will have to be further determined based on differentiating particular
patterns manifested on a particular patient.[39] In addition, a correctly diagnosed
illness can offer information on the possible direction of illness development
so that a physician can anticipate the rise of certain problems in the course of
treatment and take the anticipated problems into consideration in designing
therapeutic strategies. For example, "stagnation illness" (*yuzheng* 郁证 or *yubing*
郁病) includes various syndrome patterns that are perceived as resulting from
disordered emotional or mental activities. It normally starts with the liver *qi*
stagnation (*ganqi yujie* 肝气郁结), which could lead to restrained functions of
the spleen (*ganyu yi pi* 肝郁抑脾) and eventually to the depletion of the heart
(*xinyin kuixu* 心阴亏虚). When a problem is classified as a stagnation illness,
although the current manifestations indicate that only the liver system is affected, an experienced doctor would consider the anticipated problems with the
spleen or the heart in deciding on therapeutics.[40]

From the clinical point of view of "*kanbing*" (looking at illness), an illness
name also functions as a topic or a point of focus that both the patient and
the doctor are oriented to while the doctor engages in studying various manifestations, tracing complicated connections and mapping out the pathological conditions. When the doctor translates the patient's complaint of "unable
to sleep" (*shuibuzhao jiao* 睡不着觉) into an illness name "insomnia" (*bumei*
不寐), he or she makes the "topic" medically relevant and makes available all
the professional "comments" relevant to the topic, including accumulated experience (*jingyan* 经验) of the past. A *zhongyi* illness name then is used as a
resource rather than a constraint. By bringing an illness name into the diagnostic process, the physician juxtaposes the current case with the similar ones
that were encountered and recorded by other scholar-physicians and derives
an appropriate treatment strategy for the concrete case at hand through his
personal synthesis based on all the information available to him. For instance,
when a pathological manifestation is identified as "the running pig *qi* illness"
(*bentunqi* 奔豚气) characterized by an experienced sensation of *a* gust of *qi*,
like a running pig, dashing from the lower abdomen up to the throat, usually accompanied with a severe stomach ache, the physician then connects this
particular case with a pool of relevant discursive comments and practical treat-
ments. My *zhongyi* teacher brought in discussions of "*bentunqi*" (running pig *qi*

illness) in *Jingkui Yaolue* 金匮要略 (Essentials) of Golden Casket[41] to impress his student doctors about using the classic knowledge as resources to facilitate one's clinical reasoning. Yet the identification of an illness as *bentunqi* does not oblige the doctor to use Zhongjing's running pig *qi* formula (*bentun tang* 奔豚汤) or "strengthened cinnamon formula" (*guizhi jia gui tang* 桂枝加桂汤). The determination of an actual therapy depends on the physician's own analysis and synthesis of the information based on the particular case and patient.[42]

In this sense, *qingzhi bing* (emotion-related disorders), sometimes called "*shenzhi bing*" 神志病 (mind-related disorder)[43], should not be understood as a particular disease entity but a *zhongyi* illness term that groups various recurrent manifestation patterns that are viewed as typically having an excess of the seven emotions as the illness factors (*bingyin* 病因) and disturbed flow of *qi* as the illness mechanism (*bingji* 病机).

The categorization of *qingzhi bing* reflects the inconsistency and plurality of *zhongyi* classification of illness names (*bing ming*). Some *zhongyi* texts include the illnesses such as *dian* 癫 (apathy/despondence) and *kuang* 狂 (maniac/madness) in the category of *qingzhi* disorders since these illnesses are perceived as mental/emotional/physiological abnormalities that also originated from disordered activities of the seven emotions.[44] Others categorize *dian* and *kuang* separately from *qingzhi* disorders.[45] In the textbook *Zhongyi Internal Medicine* (*Zhongyi Neikexue* 中医内科学), *qingzhi* is not used explicitly as an illness name, but *yuzheng* (stagnation illness) and *diankuang* (apathy and madness) are listed as separate illnesses.[46] However, in the chapter on *yuzheng*, other *qingzhi* disorders such as *meiheqi* 梅核气 (the plum pit *qi* syndrome) and *bentunqi* (running pig syndrome) are listed and discussed. In other words, *yuzheng* is used in a broader sense to refer to typical *qingzhi* disorders in general.

I can certainly see the logic of this arrangement since the boundaries among *yuzheng* (stagnation illness), *meiheqi* (the plum pit *qi* syndrome), and other *qingzhi*-related disorders are not clear-cut. They are seen as specific illness conditions observed and summarized at a specific point of a pathological process related to disordered emotions. *Yu* (stagnation of *qi*) frequently dominates the initial stage of this process. As has been repeatedly demonstrated, in the Chinese world of constant change and transformation, differences are seen more in terms of position in time and place. In fact, even *dian* (apathy/despondence) and *kuang* (maniac/madness) are not essentially different from *yuzheng*. The stagnant *qi* may proceed to produce pathological phlegm that could "blind the heart-mind" (*mengbi xinshen* 蒙蔽心神) and cause "chaotic mind" (*shenzhi niluan* 神志逆乱) and "agitation and restlessness" (*kuangzao buning* 狂躁不宁) characteristics of *diankuang*. Therefore, in the coming chapter I choose to focus on *yu* 郁 (stagnation of *qi*) as the core meaning of *qingzhi* disorders and show how other meanings in connection to *yu* arise when the syndrome manifestation changes. The next chapter describes various clinical manifestations of *yu*-related patterns of *qingzhi* disorders.

Manifestations of *Yu* (Stagnation)

During the course of my clinical observation, I started to associate the specific patterns of disturbed *qi* movement, particularly the liver *qi* stagnation (*ganqi yujie* 肝气郁结) with *qingzhi* disorders (see tables 5.2 and 5.3 for reference). It is also abbreviated as "*ganyu*." Sometimes it is referred to directly as "stagnation syndrome" (*yuzheng* 郁证). A typical description of *ganqi yujie* syndrome in a *zhongyi* textbook starts:

> [Main symptoms]: dark complexion, low spirit, miserable facial expression, depressed mood, no aspiration, pessimistic, withdrawn, avoiding talking with people, feeling lonely, aversion to loud sound, restless, short tempered and feeling of fullness and swelling in the chest, lower abdomen discomfort and pain, pressure in stomach area, poor digestion and no appetite, irregular bowel movement, (female) irregular menstruation, menstruation pain and feelings of breasts swelling and pain, tongue coating thin and white sometimes with grease, pulse strung.[1]

The clusters of the symptoms are presented as having their origins in human conditions, as the author's analysis goes on to show:

> This syndrome pattern originates frequently from one's disappointment in getting what one seeks (*suoqiu busui* 所求不遂), or one's failure to achieve his/her goals (*zhiyi buda* 志意不达), or from wrongs with no channel of redress (*yinqu nanshen* 隐曲难申), thoughts and feelings tangled up without a solution (*quyi nanjie* 曲意难解), or from being constantly worried, sad, and pensive (*youchou silu* 忧愁思虑), or from anger and indignation (*fenmen naonu* 愤懑恼怒).

These illness factors, in fact, accompany *qingzhi* disorders in general. Zhang Jingyue (1562–1639) wrote that an illness of stagnation caused by excessive worries and concerns (*youyu* 忧郁) has everything to do with daily worries and concerns relating to food, clothing, and personal interest.[2] This chapter focuses particularly on *yu* as the core meaning of *qingzhi* disorders and explores various clinical manifestations associated with the pathological condition of stagnation of emotions.

UNDERSTANDING THE CONCEPT OF "YU" (STAGNATION)

As discussed in chapter 3, a persistent tendency in Chinese thinking is to see motion and change (*dong* 动) as generative of "the myriad things" of the world. In this world of ceaseless transformations, health is maintained by orderly flow and exchanges of the life forces of *jing* 精 (fine essence), *qi* 气 (life/vital energy), and *xue* 血 (blood). According to Chinese medical theory, when the orderliness of bodily processes is upset (*dong shi qi chang* 动失其常)—for example, what is supposed to go up fails to go up and what is supposed to move down fails to move down—the physiological circulations would be obstructed, and illness would arise. Seven unchecked emotive activities are the common reasons for the loss of dynamically maintained equilibrium of human physiology.

> *Neijing: Suwen (39):* "When thinking excessively (*si* 思), thoughts are stored in the heart, concentrated in one place, whereby the orthopathic *qi* stops moving and becomes static. That's why *qi* is congealed (*jie* 结)."[3]

> *Neijing: Lingshu:* "When sad and worried (*youchou* 忧愁), passage of *qi* closes and its movement stops."

> *Zhubing Yuanhou Lun:* "*Qi* congestion illness (*jieqi bing* 结气病) is produced by sadness and worry (*yousi* 忧思). When thoughts weigh in the heart, spirit stops, *qi* gets stuck and therefore congealed inside."[4]

> *Gujing Yitong Daquan:* "*Yu* refers to the blockage of the seven emotions, which leads to congestion of *qi*. Once *qi* gets stagnated, it gradually turns into various pathological forms."[5]

Apparently, *yu*, and *jie*, in earlier *zhongyi* texts, refers frequently to the pathological condition of *qi* congestion and stagnation resulting from an excess of the seven emotions.[6] Descriptions and concepts of illnesses related to emotion-induced *qi* stagnation and congestion can be found in the earliest *zhongyi* classics. The plum pit *qi* illness (*meiheqi* 梅核气) discussed in Zhang Zhongjing's *Jingkui Yaolue* (Essentials of Golden Cabinet), refers to the pathological condition related to stagnation of emotions (*qingzhi yujie* 情志郁结) that results in *qi* congestion and consequently coagulation of phlegm. This illness is still commonly present in contemporary *zhongyi* clinics. A similar disorder is called "*qi* congestion illness" (*jieqibing* 结气病 or *qibing* 气病) in *Zhubing Yuanhou Lun* (On the Sources and Origins of Various Illnesses).[7]

Yu became a more focused concern of the Danxi School of medical approach originated by the famous Yuan scholar-physician Zhu Danxi (1281–1358), who emphasized "the internal injuries" (*neishang* 内伤) as causes of illness and was well known for treating various difficult illnesses (*za bing* 杂病) such as *yu*.

He maintained that "human illnesses largely result from *yu*."[8] He divided the *yu* disorder into six subtypes. They are "stagnation of *qi*" (*qiyu* 气郁), "stagnation of dampness" (*shiyu* 湿郁), "stagnation of heat" (*reyu* 热郁), "stagnation of mucus" (*tanyu* 痰郁), "stagnation of blood" (*xueyu* 血郁), and "stagnation of food" (*shiyu* 食郁).[9] Although the six types show different syndrome configurations, they are related temporally. Typically, stagnation of *qi* is the initial problem that progresses into other types of *yu*. Wang Andao (1332–91), a student of Zhu Danxi, following the Neijing language, classifies *yu* disorder into five patterns according to their associations with five transformative phases (*wuxing* 五行), thus connecting *yu* with the five visceral systems. Wang named them "wood stagnation" (*muyu* 木郁) manifested in the liver system, "fire stagnation" (*huoyu* 火郁) manifested in the heart system, "earth stagnation" (*tuyu* 土郁) manifested in the spleen system, "metal stagnation" (*jinyu* 金郁) manifested in the lung system, and "water stagnation" (*shuiyu* 水郁) manifested in the kidney system and also talked about different methods to release different types of stagnations.[10] Danxi's other student, Dai Sigong (1324–1405), followed Danxi's classification of six types of *yu* but argued that stagnation of *qi* in the spleen and stomach system were most common. He devoted a chapter to discussing *yubing* 郁病 (*yu* illness).[11] The disorder of *yu* was understood by physicians of the Danxi school in a much broader term, namely, obstructions of the flow of *qi* in any forms and in all visceral systems caused by any pathogenic factors including excessive emotions.

During the Ming and Qing periods, discussions of *yubing* or *yuzheng* tended to center more on emotions as illness factors. Zhao Xianke (1573–1644), a Ming physician, who also had a chapter on *yubing* in his book, *Yiguan* 医贯 (On Uniformity of Medicine), felt it necessary to argue against the narrow definition of *yu*. He argued that *yu* should not be interpreted narrowly as "stagnation of sadness/worries" (*youyu zhi yu* 忧郁之郁). He insisted on a broader definition of *yu* as simply "blockage" (*butong* 不通), which included "stagnation of sadness/worries" (*youyu* 忧郁), an illness of the seven emotions (*qiqing zhi bing* 七情之病).[12] Zhang Jiebin (1560–1640), another Ming scholar-physician, was the first to make a distinction between "stagnations originating from physiological disorders" (*yin bing er yu* 因病而郁) and "illness due to stagnation of emotions" (*yin yu er bing* 因郁而病),or simply "stagnation of emotions" (*qingzhi zhi yu* 情志之郁). Zhang pointed out that since the latter originated from the heart-mind (*zong you hu xin* 总由乎心), drugs (*yaoshi* 药石) alone might not be able to dissolve the stagnation.[13] Miu Xiyong (1546–1527), a later Ming scholar-physician, also cautioned about the limitations of using only drugs to treat illnesses resulting from excessive seven emotions. He argued that even if the herbal remedy could help unblock the stagnant *qi* and activate the circulation of the blood, the problem would relapse if the illness of the heart-mind (*xin bing* 心病) persisted. He suggested using "medicine of the heart-mind" (*xin yao* 心药) to treat "an illness of the heart-mind" (*xin bing*), that is, "use thought to dispel/change thought and use reason to dissolve/transform emotions" (*yi shi*

qian shi 以识遣识; *yi li qian qing* 以理遣情).[14] Ye Tianshi (1666–1745), in his
chapter on *yuzheng*, made a clear remark that healing *yuzheng* "all depends on
the patient's ability to transform emotions and change personalities" (*quan zai
bing zhe neng yi qing yi xing* 全在病者能移情易性).[15]

Apparently, once *qingzhi zhi yu* (stagnation of emotions) was separate from
other forms of stagnation disorders, affective aspects of *yu* began to receive
more focused attention, not just in the description of illness factors (*bing yin* 病
因), illness mechanisms (*bing ji* 病机), but also symptoms and signs (*bing zheng*
病症) and therapeutic methods (*zhifa* 治法). At least in the late Ming period,
the semantics of *yu* gradually acquired a distinctive affective dimension of sadness, unhappiness, and melancholy. When Western psychology and psychiatric medicine was introduced to China, "stagnation of sadness/worries" (*youyu*)
was used to translate the Western concepts of "depression" and "melancholy."
The commonly used psychiatric disease name of depression (*yiyu* 抑郁) also
has the character '*yu*' in its Chinese translation. As the *zhongyi* concept of *yu*
was appropriated for modern use, the phenomenological sense of "blockage of
flow" (*butong* 不通) inherited in the Chinese concept of *yu* would inevitably be
slipped into the Chinese commonsensical understanding of depression (*youyu*
or *yiyu*). Conversely, the modern use of *yu* as a psychological and psychiatric
term has definitely influenced its meaning in contemporary *zhongyi* discourse
and practice and reinforced its *zhongyi* conception as *qingzhi* related, thus allowing a possible referential connection between a *qingzhi* disorder and a Western psychological disorder. *Yuzheng* in contemporary *zhongyi* textbooks and
practices refers predominantly to the narrower sense of *qingzhi zhi yu* (stagnation of emotions).[16] In today's *zhongyi* textbooks, *yuzheng* is used to include a
group of illnesses and patterns of syndrome that originate from "the blocked
flow of emotions" (*qingzhi bu shu* 情志不舒) and "the impeded *qi* mechanism
(*qiji yuzhi* 气机郁结).

CLINICAL CONFIGURATIONS OF YU (STAGNATION)

In *zhongyi* clinics, as discussed previously, differentiation of patterns is the central focus of the clinical work and is directly relevant to the determination of
therapeutic methods. Often an illness name, such as *yuzheng* is implied in the
process of differentiation of patterns (*bianzheng*) and therapy determination
(*zhifa*). *Yuzheng*, like all other *zhongyi* illnesses, is perceived as a disordered
psychophysiological process, and hence attention is always given to the temporal and spatial qualities of the dynamic relations of the symptoms. As shown
in table 6.1, *yuzheng* in general may appear as various pattern configurations
and may even acquire different illness names. On the one hand, these pattern
configurations can be seen as different stages of the same illness process. From
qi stagnation, to fire, to phlegm, and to depletion, we can easily recognize the
temporal and spatial continuities among these patterns. On the other hand,
they are unique configurations of particular social and psychophysiological

Table 6.1   *Zheng* (Patterns) and *Qingzhi* Disorders

Zheng 证 (Syndrome Types)	Affected Visceral Systems	Condition of qi and blood	Main Symptoms	Relevant Illnesses
The liver *qi* stagnation	Liver and Stomach	Stagnation of *qi*	Depressed emotion, thoracic fullness, and pain, vexation, irritability	*Yuzheng* (*qi* stagnation syndrome)
Stagnant liver *qi* turned into fire	Liver, Heart, Stomach	Stagnation of *qi* and congestion of blood	restlessness, insomnia, bad temper, bitter mouth, dry throat, tongue red, coating yellow	*Yuzheng* *Fanzao bumei* (Insomnia due to vexation)
Qi stagnant and congestion of phlegm	Liver, Heart, Spleen	Stagnation of *qi*	depressed mood, chest pressure, emotionless expression, feeling of blockage in the throat	*Yuzheng* *Dian* or *kuang* (madness) *Zangzao* (visceral agitation)
The heart *yin* depletion	Heart, Lung	Depletion of blood and *yin* fluids	headache, dizziness, palpitation, decreased memory, restlessness, unstable emotions	*Zangzao* *Baihe bing* (hundred confusions) *Beidie* (inferior syndrome)
Depletion in both the heart and the spleen	Heart, Spleen	Depletion of both *qi* and blood	yellowish facial complexion, weeping, headache and dizziness, poor appetite, insomnia	*Yuzheng* *Zangzao* *Beidie*
Yin depletion leading to "depleted" fire	Heart, Liver, Kidney	Depletion of the liver blood and kidney *jing*	red facial complexion, red eyed, unclear vision, excessive dreaming, irritable, unstable emotions	*Yuzheng* *Baihebing*

environments of the time that call for different names and different therapies. Emotion stagnation affects the three visceral systems of the liver, the spleen, and the heart most frequently.

The patterns listed in table 6.1 are by no means all of the configurations that are pertinent to *qingzhi* or *yu* disorders, but they are the most common ones that I encountered during my clinical observations of a particular physician who is known as especially adept at treating various *yu* illnesses.[17] The cases I present below demonstrate both the shared clinical knowledge of treating *yu* disorders by *zhongyi* physicians in the past and present and the particular physician's experience, styles of doctoring, and personal synthesis of various sources of knowledge in his approach to emotion-related illnesses.

Occasionally, *qingzhi bing* or *yuzheng* is directly referred to in the clinics, but very often it is implied in a particular pattern of syndrome manifestation and unfolded in the process of pattern differentiation and therapy determination. Then, for the researcher, recognizing a *qingzhi*-related disorder itself is an interpretive process involving the making out of meaningful connections among symptoms (*zheng* 症), syndrome patterns (*zhenghou* 证候), therapeutic principles (*zhifa* 治法), herbal formulas (*fangyao* 方药), and references to the materials of the medical classics, and most of all involving the understanding of clinical communications between the doctor and the patient.

Ganqi Yujie (the Liver *Qi* Stagnation)

As discussed above, clinically *yuzheng* (stagnation illness) starts when imbalanced emotions upset the *qi* circulation. Once excessive anger causes the *qi*

Table 6.2 Distribution of *Qingzhi* Disorders According to *Zheng* (Patterns) Among 150 Patients

Differentiation of Zheng (Syndromes)	No. of cases	% of the cases	Liver	Heart	Spleen	Kidney	Gall Bladder
The liver *qi* stagnation	23	15	23	7	4		1
Stagnant *qi* turned into fire	11	7	11	3	3		
Qi stagnant and phlegm congestion	28	19	23	22		1	
The heart *yin* depletion	27	18	1	27	2	1	
Both heart and spleen depletion	17	11		17	17		
Yin depletion and depleted fire	30	20	9	23		10	
Other	14	9	4	5	1	2	7
Total	150	100	71	104	27	14	8

Differentiation of zheng is based on the first diagnosis as qingzhi related.

movement to reverse and to block the circulation, it hurts the liver system first since the liver functions to disperse *qi*. It is very likely that the accumulated stagnant *qi* in the liver system encroaches on the stomach system (*ganqi fan wei* 肝气犯胃). Therefore, the manifestations also include the symptoms pertaining to the spleen and the stomach system, such as "feelings of pressure in the stomach area and frequent hiccups," "abdominal gas and loss of appetite," "vomiting," and "abnormal bowel movement." For a female patient, since *qi* is the driving force of the movement of blood in circulation (*qi wei xue zhi shuai* 气为血之帅), and when *qi* gets stagnant, the blood tends to congeal, the patient may experience disordered menstruation. *Yuzheng*, in its narrow sense, refers particularly to the illness manifestation at this stage of liver *qi* stagnation. The temporal and spatial dimension is marked by an extension from the liver system to the stomach system and to the congestion of the blood. In my clinical observation, *ganyu* was a frequent initial manifestation of the *qingzhi* disorder. As shown in table 6.2, among the 150 patients who suffered *qingzhi* disorders, 15 percent suffered purely from liver *qi* stagnation. But, if we consider the cases of liver *qi* stagnation combined with liver fire and pathological phlegm, the percentage of the liver *qi* stagnation is 41 percent.

In my first illustrative case, a 53-year-old woman came to the clinic originally for a headache. She was diagnosed as suffering from a heat-related disorder and was prescribed medicine to nourish the blood and clear heat (*yangxue qingre* 养血清热). She came back a week later. She looked even more depressed and unhappy. She told the doctor that after taking six bags of herbal medicine, her headache seemed to improve, but she felt *qi* pressure in her heart (*xinli bieqi* 心里憋气), and there was a sense of blockage (*fadu* 发堵) in her chest. She gave long sighs as if by doing this she could help herself release some of the *qi* stuck inside her chest. She also had experienced a bloated stomach and abdomen and complained of heart vexation (*xinfan* 心烦) and bad temper. While talking, she broke into tears. She began to tell the doctor that she had moved to Beijing from Shandong province in 1985 following her husband's transfer. She had not had a permanent job since. She regretted moving to Beijing. In Shandong she was a high school teacher and her work was meaningful and respected by others. Now she worked as a temporary elevator operator. She felt her life was completely meaningless. Her mother had died several months before at the age of 89. After that, she cried almost every day. Her son had been admitted into Beijing College of Political Sciences, and she hated the idea that her son was going to study something related to politics, which, she thought, was useless, empty, and potentially dangerous. She wanted him to be an engineer.

The doctor proceeded with his examination while listening to the patient. The patient's pulse was heavy and thin (*chenxi* 沉细), the color of her tongue was dark, and the coating was white and thin. According to the syndrome differentiation, the patient suffered liver *qi* stagnation (*ganqi yujie*). Therapeutic principle was determined to disperse the liver system and revitalize the flow of *qi* and to dissolve the stagnancy and eliminate vexation (*shugan liqi, jieyu chufan* 疏肝理气, 解郁除烦). The patient was prescribed the modified Chaihu Shugansan 柴胡舒肝散 (the formula of bupleuri for dispersing the stagnant liver *qi*)." Five more herbs were added to the original formula.

The patient's illness was obviously *qingzhi* related and had a clear social origin. The first time she came in, she mainly complained about the headache and the sensation of heat in five hearts (*wuxin fanre* 五心烦热). The tip of her tongue was red, and the coating was yellow. All symptoms pointed to heat damage. On the second visit, the symptoms were different, and the whole pathological configuration changed. Therefore, a new diagnosis was required. The doctor commented that the patient's illness came from a situation in which everything was going against her heart's will (*zhushi bushunxin* 诸事不顺心), and therefore her heart-emotion was constrained (*xinqing yayi* 心情压抑), which caused the impeded *qi* mechanism leading to *qi* accumulation in the liver system. I expressed doubts that the herbal medicine would be effective, since we already knew that the patient's problem resulted from her social situations and emotional experiences. The doctor responded positively without hesitation: "It will definitely work" (*kending guanyong* 肯定管用). He explained that the herbs help attune the bodily functions. Once the bodily functions improve, the symptoms will recede, the patient's bodily experience will be altered, and the patient's heart-emotion (*xinqing*) will certainly change for the better. For *zhongyi* doctors, the symptoms, such as blockage in the heart, pressure in the chest, and empty-fullness (*piman* 痞满) in the stomach are not imagined or secondary to anything. They are real experiences that can be treated by taking herbal medicine. I personally heard many times that a patient came back to the clinic and claimed, "My heart-emotion is feeling much better" (*xinqing hao duo le* 心情好多了). The doctor also agreed that the patient suffering from a *qingzhi* disorder tended to relapse. "Once you see a patient coming for treatment and recovered, and then coming back again, you immediately know that there must be problems in her social environment. But a doctor can only do as much as he can."

Doctors do much more than just prescribe herbal medicine. In the above case, the doctor was engaging the patient in a conversation while examining her and composing a herbal formula. He showed his sympathy with the patient and agreed with her that it was not always good to give up everything just to get into Beijing. He then went on to say that there were still thousands of people on the waiting lists for a residential quota in order to move into Beijing, and she would be considered lucky by those who were still waiting. When the patient talked about the death of her mother, he asked about the age of her mother. The doctor then said that the mother had lived a "long life" (*gaoshou* 高寿), was something, in the ancient times, worth celebrating. As for the patient's complaint about her son's choice of school, the doctor commented that everybody, even the patient's son, has a piece of his own sky above his head and she could not live for him. He spoke of his experience with his own son who, against his will, insisted on going into business. Finally, he said jokingly to the patient,

Who knows, someday your son might became an important political figure." The patient could not help but smile.

QIYU HUAHUO 气郁化火
(STAGNANT QI TRANSFORMED INTO FIRE)

According to the *zhongyi* physiology, once the stagnant *qi* is accumulated and condenses for some time without an open passage to channel it out, it turns into fire (*yu jiu hua huo* 郁久化火). Different symptom configurations reflect this physiological change. Since liver fire tends to flare upward, the patient may experience headaches and dizziness, and the facial complexion tends to be slightly red. Since the liver is connected with the gall bladder, the fire together with the *qi* of the gall bladder moves upward and the patient may experience dry throat and bitter mouth. With the wood (the liver system) losing its elasticity (ability to extend) (*tiaoda* 条达), the patient may be short tempered and irritable. As the liver fire disturbs the functions of the stomach, the patient may also experience gastric discomfort with acid regurgitation (*caoza tunsuan* 嘈咂吞酸) and dry stool. The liver fire also extends to the heart system (which is next to the wood phase in the *wuxing* production sequence) and disturbs the heart-mind (*xinshen* 心神), and the symptoms of vexation and agitation appear. The tongue is red, the coating yellow, and the pulse strung and fast. All these symptoms show that the stagnation of *qi* has transformed into fire. However, excessive anger and rage damage the liver systems directly and may lead to liver fire without an initial period of liver *qi* stagnation. Some clinicians see this syndrome as a prelude to more serious mental illness, since if the condition worsens, it can lead to "craziness" (*kuangluan wuzhi* 狂乱无知).[18]

In my second illustrative case, a woman of 25 years old, was married several months before she came to the clinic. She complained that she had disturbed sleep. It was difficult for her to fall sleep, and she woke up easily. She was irritable and bad tempered (*piqida* 脾气大). She said she did not know why she had such a "big fire" (*huoqida* 火气大) and became angry so easily. She had an urge to break things and had already smashed the mirror and the cassette player at home. In reply to the doctor's question whether she felt wronged (*weiqu* 委屈) and tended to cry a lot, the patient said that she had seldom cried before she was married, but found herself constantly crying after she was married. She complained about her husband's narrow-mindedness (*xiao xinyan* 小心眼) and said that her husband found fault with her over trifling things. The doctor told her that insomnia was not her problem; the problem was her vexation. Her case belonged to the category of insomnia caused by vexation of the heart-mind (*xinfan bude mian* 心烦不得眠), so the treatment should focus on her heart-mind problem. The doctor then asked about the patient's background, such as if she was the youngest in her family and if she was considered to be spoiled (*jiaoqi* 娇气). The patient was actually the oldest child with a younger sister and a brother. She also denied that she was spoiled but said before her marriage she was generally considered nice and good tempered (*piqi hao* 脾气 好). She broke into tears. At the end of the consultation, the doctor referred the patient to me, saying that she should talk with me and that I was doing research on emotion-related problems.

The patient's complexion was slightly red. She had a bitter mouth and dry throat, suggesting the liver fire and the gall-bladder *qi* moving up. The tip of her tongue was red, but the coating was white, which did not totally support the other symptoms. Her pulse was strung and fast. Her syndrome was differentiated as "the stagnant liver *qi* turning into fire" (*ganyu huahuo* 肝郁化火), though the doctor pointed out that some of the symptoms did not totally support the syndrome differentiation. For example, the white coating of the tongue did not support the presence of the fire. However, the doctor, in consideration of the whole symptom configuration, came to the conclusion that the stagnant *qi* had just started to turn into fire. He explained that the patient's main problem was *ganyu* that had already shown the sign of fire. Therefore, the therapeutic principle was to disperse the liver *qi*, dissolve the stagnation, and eliminate vexation (*shugan, jieyu, chufan* 疏肝解郁除烦). The patient was prescribed *xiaoyao san* 逍遥散 (xiaoyao powder), with two other herbs added to strengthen the function of eliminating vexation.

In this case, the patient and the doctor both recognized that the patient's suffering was not a simple physical discomfort. The patient complained mainly about her insomnia but pointed to her anger and her dissatisfaction with her marriage as the source of her suffering. The doctor's questions were also directed to the social origin of the illness and he concluded that insomnia was not the problem, but *ganyu* (the liver qi stagnation). Liver *qi* stagnation is understood as an emotion disorder coming from the blocked circulation in an emotional, social, and physical sense. When this *qi* is blocked for a period of time, it starts to turn into liver fire that manifests itself in a person in the form of excessive anger and irascibility. This *zhongyi* concept has long become "commonsense." In everyday language, when somebody is irritable and tends to become angry easily, she is said to be "having a big fire *qi*" (*huoqi da*)or "having a big liver fire" (*ganhuo wang* 肝火旺).

The patient and I walked out of the clinic together and found a relatively quiet corner in the waiting area for a conversation. It was not a strict interview format. My role as an anthropologist at the moment was dubious. I was incorporated into the clinical process, more to listen and offer my support than to elicit answers to anthropological questions. When I came back to the clinical room and supplied the doctor with more detailed information about the patient, he said that the *zhongyi* tradition has encouraged the doctor to consider information that goes beyond the immediate physical symptoms. For example, *Neijing: Suwen* (77) emphasizes that a doctor, when treating a patient, has to take into consideration changes in the natural environment (*tianshi* 天时), the social and economic situation (*renshi* 人事), and the visceral (*zangxiang* 脏象) and pulse (*maise* 脉色) manifestations. It is considered a mistake (*guo* 过) for the doctor not to enquire about the patient's social background and emotional changes, such as if the person has experienced changes from a high status to a lower status, financial changes, ambition for power or sudden joy, sadness, or anger. Traditionally, such information was more readily accessible to the doctor, who, usually, was a knowledgeable and well-respected member of the community and was routinely called to the patient's home to treat the patient. However, the doctor said that today's *zhongyi* practice is organized in a way different from what it used to be and that a doctor has to make a deliberate effort to get personal information beyond a patient's immediate illness concerns. Yet a modern *zhongyi* doctor is cautious about asking sensitive questions. He or she depends more on personal experience and intuition as well as communication skills to understand the patient's situation. In addition, unlike a typical psychologist, who depends on insight into the patient's intrapsychic conflicts for effective treatment, a *zhongyi* doctor does not need to know every detail of the patient's personal life and social relations to differentiate a syndrome or design an herbal formula.

Qizhi Tanyu 气滞痰郁 (*Qi* Stagnation Leading to Congestion of Phlegm)

The syndrome is also known as "congestion of phlegmatic *qi*" (*tanqi yujie* 痰气郁结). When the liver *qi* is stagnant, it encroaches on the spleen system that belongs to the earth phase. It interferes with the spleen's functions of transforming and transmitting (*yunhua* 运化) nutrients and water throughout the body. The dampness is then accumulated to form phlegm, which further blocks the movement of *qi* in the body. This particular doctor offered a different explanation for the phenomenon of phlegmatic *qi* congestion. His logic was that *ganyu* leads to fire, which dries up the bodily fluid (*jinye* 津液) and turns it into relatively thick phlegm. This pathological process is known as "burning the bodily fluid into phlegm" (*zhuojin huatan* 灼津化痰), which points to two physiological consequences. One is the potential depletion of vital fluid, which will lead to the condition of *yin* depletion; the other is the blockage of circulation which is much harder to treat than the stagnation of *qi*.

When the blockage formed by congealed phlegm is above the thoracic area, the patient experiences the sensation of an alien object stuck in the throat, which cannot be spit out or swallowed. This manifestation type has acquired the rather vivid illness name, "the plum pit *qi*" (*meiheqi* 梅核气). This illness term was first used by the Han dynasty physician, Zhang Zhongjing to refer to an illness that was later included in *yu* disorders. During my clinical observation, I noticed two cases of the plum pit *qi*. One such case was particularly interesting. The patient frequently cleared her throat and found a thread of blood in her phlegm. She feared that there was something growing in her throat. The doctor, after examining her, told her that there was nothing growing in her throat and that her illness was actually "*qi* congestion" (*qi bing*) originating from anger (*shengqi* 生气).[19] Hearing this, the patient agreed completely with the doctor that her illness all started from her resentment about her husband's intimate relationship with one of his female colleagues. She asked the doctor to tell her husband exactly what he had told her when her husband called to inquire about the clinical result. In a sense, by involving the doctor in an interaction with the family members, the patient successfully employed the doctor's help in manipulating her social relations. The patient later told me admiringly that the doctor was so experienced (*you jingyan* 有经验) that he could immediately detect what the real problem was.

If the heteropathic *qi* of phlegm continues to block the passage, it may finally disturb "the clear openings" (*shangrao qingqiao* 上扰清窍) and "blind the heart-mind" (*mengbi xinshen* 蒙蔽心神). This particular stage of the pathological course is called "the phlegm blocking the opening of the heart-mind" (痰迷心窍). The symptom configuration then may include "depressed mood," "indifferent expressions," "quietness and motionlessness," "illogical speech," "self-talk," and "unpredictable changes of mood between happiness and anger." This manifestation of syndrome configuration is also known as "*dian* 癫," characterized by quietness, absentmindedness, incoherent language, and a perpetual "happy facial expression." *Dian* is also discussed in relation to "*kuang* 狂," characterized by "loudness and restlessness," "violent behavior," and being "full of anger." These two illnesses cannot be strictly separated in symptoms and are able to transform into each other. Therefore, *dian* and *kuang* are sometimes discussed together as one illness, *diankuang*.[20]

Since the mental and emotional disturbance of *dian* is serious enough to be recognized as full-blown mental illness (*jingshen bing* 精神病), in many textbooks *dian* is not included in the discussions of *qingzhi* (emotion-related) disorders.[21] Yet the difference between a *qingzhi* disorder and *dian* is seen mainly as a difference of "*du*" (degree, position).[22] Patients suffering from *dian* do come to see doctors of *zhongyi*. During my entire period of clinical observation, there were only two cases for which the doctor used *dian* as the illness name. In one case, a young female patient visited the clinic with her husband. Throughout the interview, the patient remained emotionless and motionless. She did not say a single word. Her husband did all the talking. The patient was a manager of a sweater factory. She had signed six contracts with clients within several months and had become extremely worried about her factory's ability to fulfill the contracts. She had developed insomnia and was constantly restless. The symptoms were getting worse. She was suicidal, weeping, and became increasingly absentminded, to the point that she was not able to work at all. The doctor's diagnosis was "the opening of the heart-mind blocked by congealed phlegm" (*tan mi xin qiao*). He added, "according to *zhongyi*, this is *dian*." This patient did not return to the clinic after her first visit. No further information on this patient was obtained.

The second case was a 22-year-old male university student. He came to the clinic three times, showing steady improvement each time. The first time he came, he did not talk at all. He was expressionless and withdrawn. His mother did most of the talking. According to his mother, he was a student in a prestigious university in Beijing. He was traumatized and became ill.[23] He experienced delusions, was depressed, and wanted to kill himself. The doctor said that in *zhongyi* language, the patient was suffering *dian* illness or *tan mi xinqiao*. The third time, I saw him, though he still looked passive, he talked about his illness himself and told the doctor that he had felt an improvement. At least he could sleep for several hours at a time. Other cases that were related to "heteropathic phlegm that disturbed the heart-mind" (*tan rao xinshen* 痰扰心神) were not as serious as *tan mi xinqiao*. Therefore, the doctor did not explicitly talk about those cases as *dian*.

In the third illustrative case, a 50-year-old man accompanied by his wife came to see the doctor. He was the last patient of that morning. He seemed very reluctant to come into the clinic, and his wife literally pushed him into the consulting room. He looked melancholy and diffident. His voice was soft and low. He complained about dizziness, heart-mind not together (*jingshen huanghu* 精神恍惚), difficulty sleeping, thinking too much, suspiciousness (*duoyi* 多疑), and lack of confidence (*zuoshi weisuo* 做事畏缩). He said that he created trouble for himself (*ziji gen ziji guo buqu* 自己跟自己过不去). and that he was oversensitive (*xiao xinyan* 小心眼). He thought his problem started with worry over the health of his son, who was diagnosed as having myocarditis just before the patient had left home on a performance tour (he was a musician). He was worried about his son and called home almost every day. He was self-reproachful and felt guilty for his son's illness. His wife added that the patient had his only son at the age of 43. The patient talked about his son inheriting his own weakness of oversensitivity. He blamed himself for influencing his son's personality. He talked about his difficulty in concentration and said that he constantly made mistakes while playing on stage. He told the doctor that he found his fingers involuntarily brushing against things without control.

Syndrome differentiation pointed to liver *qi* stagnation leading to phlegm congestion. The turbidity of phlegm obscures the patient's heart-mind (*shenming* 神明). The doctor told the patient that his problem was mainly mental in nature (*jingshen xing de* 精神性的). A therapeutic treatment was set to clear the heart, disperse the phlegm, calm the mind, and stabilize the intellect (*jingxin huatan, anshen dingzhi* 清心化痰, 安神定志). He was prescribed decoction of pinelliae and magnoliae officinalis (*banxia houpu tang* 半夏厚朴汤) with several more herbs added to it to strengthen the function of eliminating the heat. The doctor thought the patient's illness showed the tendency of *dian* but not to the full extent of *dian*, but if the condition went on without appropriate treatment, the illness could develop into a serious mental disorder.

In many cases, excessive thinking and worrying (*silu guodu* 思虑过度) can be the direct cause of the syndrome of phlegm congestion. As known in *zhongyi*, thinking and worrying (*silu*) are emotions of the spleen system. When a person thinks and worries too much, the spleen system is directly affected. Dampness is collected to form the pathological phlegm, which converges with the phlegm problem caused by liver *qi* stagnation. The pathological process of *yu* up to this point demonstrates the pattern of repletion. The body's orthopathic *qi* (*zhengqi* 正气) is not yet significantly consumed, and the heteropathic *qi* (*xieqi* 邪气) is dominantly present.

Xinyin Kuixu 心阴亏虚 (the Heart *Yin* Depletion)

As can be seen from the above, when the pathological condition of the stagnation of *qi* continues, it turns into fire. The fire consumes the heart-blood (*haoshang xinxue* 耗伤心血), and the *yin* aspect of the heart becomes deplete. Once the heart *yin* blood is depleted, it is not able to nourish (*ruyang* 濡养) the heart-mind (*xinshen* 心神). The mind and spirit that reside in the viscera of the heart lose their home (*shen bu shou she* 神不守舍), and the symptoms of heart-mind uneasiness (*xinshen buning* 心神不宁), absent-mindedness (*jing-shen huanghu*), forgetfulness, insomnia, and excessive dreaming appear. Once the heart *yin* is depleted, the unchecked heart-fire rises up to disturb the heart-mind, and the patient feels upset and perturbed (*xinfan yiluan* 心烦意乱) and unable to sit still (*zuowo buan* 坐卧不安). Once heart-mind lacks nourishment, the ability to make judgments and solve problems is seriously impeded, and the patient shows slowness in response and a depressed mood. Since the depleted *yin* is not able to constrain or balance the *yang* (*yin bu lian yang* 阴不敛阳), the fire due to depleted *yin* becomes rampant (*xuhuo wangdong* 虚火妄动), and somatic manifestations appear, such as hotness in the five hearts (*wuxin fanre* 五心烦热), sweating palms, dry mouth and throat, slightly red complexion, red tongue with little coating, and thin and fast pulse.

This syndrome is also referred to in the medical classics and in present day *zhongyi* clinics as "*zangzao* 脏躁" (the visceral agitation) characterized by the symptoms of restlessness, sadness, and a tendency to weep and sigh. The illness name *zangzao* appears early in *Shanghan Zabing Lun* 伤寒杂病论 (*Discussion of Cold Damages and Various Disorders*), which describes the illness as "constantly feeling sad and weeping" (*xi beishang yuku* 喜悲伤易哭). The same author, Zhang Zhongjing, in *Jingui Yaolue* 金匮要略 (*Essentials of Golden Casket*), included *zangzao bing* in his discussion of women's illnesses: "A woman who suffers *zangzao* is sad and likes to weep, as if possessed by a spirit, and tends to yawn frequently."[24] The meaning of *zao* 躁 is fairly clear, suggesting disturbance and restlessness of emotions. There have been discussions as to what in the visceral system the character *zang* 脏 refers. Some believe that since *zangzao* was originally seen as a woman's illness, *zang* may stand for "womb" (*nuzibao* 女子胞). Others insist that it refers to the heart system, since the heart system is responsible for *shenming* (consciousness, intellect). Since *zangzao* describes a mental and emotional disturbance, *zang* must stand for the heart. This was clearly stated in *Yi Zong Jinjian* 医宗金鉴 (*Standard Collection of Medical Works*), edited by Wu Qian and others (1742): "*Zang*, refers to the heart (*xin*). When the heart is tranquil, *shén* (the mind; consciousness) is contained. When the heart system is injured by the seven emotions, it loses its peacefulness, and *shén* would become agitated and restless."[25] Yet, in actual practice, doctors tend not to limit their scope to a single visceral system. Tang Rongchuan (1846–97), a Qing physician, stated that doctors should not be restricted to a single visceral system, when the symptoms of *zao* (emotional agitation or disturbance) are obvious. "When there are symptoms of sadness and weeping as if the patient is possessed by ghosts, it is clear that the heart has been afflicted; when there are symptoms of excessive yawning and stretching, it is clear that the kidney has been affected."[26]

In modern *zhongyi* clinics, *zangzao* is found in both males and females. The patient suffering *zangzao* is described as "feeling like to walk but could not, feeling like to sleep but could not" (*yuxing bude xing, yuwo bude wo* 欲行不得行, 欲卧不得卧).

In my fourth illustrative case, a 55-year-old male patient who came across the manufactured "herb concoction to disperse stagnation and stabilize the mind" at a pharmacy tried it and found it helpful. So he came to see the doctor who developed the medicine, hoping he could be cured of the illness that had bothered him off and on for more than fifteen years. He complained that he was feeling restless (*zuowo buan* 坐卧不安) and heart-mind disturbed (*xinshen buning* 心神不宁). He had to walk outside constantly regardless of whether it was raining or snowing. He also complained that his vision was not clear and that he had a runny nose. He had difficulty in sleeping,. and often had to take sleeping pills. He first became ill during 1977 and 1978 when he was busy studying English in preparation for going abroad. He thought that his illness must have been caused by anxiety and stress. While he was talking to the doctor, his hands were trembling slightly. The teeth marks on his tongue were clearly visible, indicating the depletion of *qi* that had led to a depletion of *yin*. The coating of his tongue was yellow and thin. The pattern of syndrome was described as excessive thinking and worrying (*silu guodu*) that had injured the heart and spleen and led to heart *yin* depletion. The therapeutic indication was to replenish *yin* and nourish the blood (*ziyin yangxue* 滋阴养血) and to supplement the heart and calm the mind (*buxin anshen* 补心安神). He was prescribed *tianwang buxin dan* 天王补心丹 (king of heaven tonic for the heart-mind) with additions and subtractions, and the concoction to disperse the stagnation and to stabilize the mind to be taken before going to bed.

The patient came back again after six doses of the medicine. He felt less agitated, and his sleep had improved. By taking his pulse the doctor surmised that the stagnation was still present. Two more herbs were added to the original prescription. The doctor said that if the prescription worked, he would not change the formula. Unlike the previous discussed syndromes, in this case "the stagnation" (*yu*) was treated as a depletion syndrome. That is because when the stagnation is caused internally by the seven emotions, it starts damaging the *qi* movement, and when the stagnation continues, the illness hurts the blood and subsequently consumes the vital substance and life force.

Xinpi Liang Xu 心脾两虚 (Depletion of the Heart and the Spleen)

As the *yin* aspect of the heart is further depleted, the result can be depletion in both the heart *yin* and spleen *qi*. The depletion of the heart and the spleen can also be understood as resulting directly from the excessive emotion of "thinking/worrying" (*silu*). Since *si* directly affects the spleen system, it restrains its function to transmit and transform nutrients (the source of both *qi* and blood) and to provide nourishment to the heart. In turn, the depleted heart *yin* is not able to facilitate the function of the spleen and the stomach system. The result is that both blood that is *yin* and *qi* that is *yang* are depleted. The manifestation includes "excessive worrying and thinking" (*duosi shanlu* 多思善虑), "palpitation and fearfulness (*xinji danqie* 心悸胆怯), "insomnia and forgetfulness" (*shaomei jianwang* 少寐健忘). In fact, in *zhongyi* clinics, *bumei* (insomnia) and *xinji* (heart palpitation) are two frequent symptoms that bring the patients to the doctors. Chinese patients often complain of *xinji* and *bumei*, *two illnesses* recognized in *zhongyi*. They overlap with *qingzhi* disorders, especially with the pattern of depletion in the heart and the spleen.

In the fifth illustrative case, the patient was a 64-year-old retired male. His neighbor, a young woman, accompanied him to the clinic. The patient complained about a dry and bitter mouth. He had no appetite and no taste for food. He was in a bad mood and felt vexed all the time. He had low energy (*jingshen buhao* 精神不好) during the day. His head was heavy, and his neck was stiff, and he had sleeping problems. He had been to a biomedical doctor before he came to the *zhongyi* clinic and was given two types of tranquilizers to help him sleep. The color of his tongue was pale, and the coating was white, which indicated depletion of *qi* in the spleen. He was given herbal medicine to strengthen the spleen system. He came back after a week and told the doctor that some of his symptoms, such as dizziness and the heaviness of his head, seemed alleviated. But other symptoms, for example, his dry and bitter mouth, poor appetite, low energy, and poor sleep remained the same. He also had new symptoms—fluttering heart, palpitation, and shortness of breath—which also suggested depletion in his heart system. The tongue manifestation remained the same.

The patient had an angry and depressed look. The doctor asked him if he felt "wronged or self-pity" (*weiqu* 委屈), and the patient replied with an affirmative nod. Then the doctor said, as if to himself, that a person needs to feel grateful (*zhizu* 知足) and that everybody occupies a place in life where he was better off than some and was worse off than others. At this point, the doctor turned to the young woman standing behind and told her that she should take her father out more to let him relax (*sansan xin* 散散心). The young woman answered that she was his neighbor. The patient was living by himself. His wife had died not long ago, and his only son was abroad. Listening to the young woman's words, the patient looked even more miserable. We thought that the patient's son had settled in a foreign country and would not come back. Asking for more information, we learned that the son was sent out to work for two years and would be back in less than a year. The doctor then became more encouraging, assuring the patient that his illness was not serious and that he needed to be more active. He told the patient not to stay at home by himself dwelling on his own unhappiness but to visit neighbors (*cuancuan men* 窜窜门) and play chess (*xiaxia qi* 下下棋) or play cards (*dada pai* "打打牌").

The syndrome was described as depletion in both the heart and the spleen. The excessive *silu* (sadness and worries) directly damped his spleen function to transform and transmit vital materials of the body and led to the depletion of the heart since the spleen system failed to provide *yin* to nourish the heart. The therapeutic indication was to strengthen the spleen and replenish the *qi* (*jianpi puqi* 健脾补气) and to nourish the heart and calm the mind (*yangxin anshen* 养心安神). The patient was prescribed *guipi tang* 归脾汤 (decoction for invigorating spleen and nourishing heart).

The patient came back once more seeming a little improved. The doctor told me that the patient might not be totally healed before his son came back. He referred to the *zhongyi* saying "an illness due to emotion can only be completely cured by emotion" (*Yi qing bing zhe, fei qing bu jie* 以情病者非情不解).[27]

Yinxu Huowang 阴虚火旺 (Yin Depletion Leading to the Rampant Fire)

When the illness is prolonged, the *yin* of the visceral systems continues to be depleted. The heart *yin* is depleted, the liver *yin* is depleted, and finally the kidney *yin* is depleted. With the depleted visceral *yin*, the "false *yang*" (*fuyang* 浮阳) manifested as rampant fire arises. My *zhongyi* teacher used the metaphor of boiling water to illustrate the situation. He explained that when the water in a pot is getting less and less, we hear a louder sound and see a large amount of steam coming out of the pot as if the temperature is very high. The excessive activity inside the pot is actually due to insufficient water rather than the actual increase of the temperature intside. Similarly, when a person suffers from a chronic illness, and the visceral *yin* in various forms of vital fluids (blood, water, semen, and so on) is consumed without replenishment, there will be overexcitement of "false yang" or "fire." Since this excessive activity of fire is not caused by actual heteropathic invasion, it is also referred to as "fire of depletion" (*xuhuo* 虚火). The patient may demonstrate symptoms that suggest "liver fire or heart fire," such as a red face and eyes, agitation and anger, dizziness, palpitation, insomnia, red tongue with dry coating, dry mouth and throat, and so on. The more serious depletion involves the kidney system. According to the *wuxing* (five transformative phases) relationship, the kidney system is said to belong to the water phase and it stores *jing* 精 (vital essence) that is either inherited from one's parents or transformed from the nutrients taken into the body. The kidney is the storage of the life force and also the source of marrow (*sui* 髓)

and the brain since the brain is seen as "a sea of marrow" (*suizhihai* 髓之海). Therefore, when the depletion has drained the kidney *jing*, the patient may experience symptoms of memory decrease, excessive dreams, tinnitus, back pain, seminal emission (in males), irregular menstruation (in females), and coldness in the lower limbs. This illness configuration may have variations. It can appear as kidney water not sufficient to moisturize the liver wood (*shui bu hanmu* 水 不涵木) or as the heart fire not connected to the kidney water (*xinshen bujiao* 心肾不交). The therapeutic procedure usually involves replenishing *yin* and cleansing the heat.

In the sixth illustrative case, the patient was a 29-year-old male. He complained about difficulty sleeping during the night, fatigue and sleepiness during the day, nervousness, agitation, and abnormal sweating. His head seemed heavy and clouded. His eyes were tired, and his vision was blurred. He also had lower back discomfort. He thought that his illness had started with a routine physical examination ten months before. It was found that one of his physiological indexes was higher than normal, which indicated the possibility of hepatitis B. He had been worried about being ill with hepatitis B ever since. He said his work was stressful, involving constant business trips. Although he had been taking some manufactured Chinese medicine, the effect was little. At most he was able to sleep only four hours a day. The experience was painful, and he said he would rather have hepatitis B than his present disorder that rendered him dysfunctional and depressed. The patient's symptom configuration suggests both the unchecked "empty fire" that disturbed the heart-mind and depletion of the liver and kidney *yin*. The doctor explained to the patient that his excessive obsession with his *shenti* (health) actually led to the stagnation of *qi*, which in turn was transformed into fire that consumed and harmed the visceral *yin*.

The syndrome differentiation was *yin* depletion leading to rampant "empty fire." The therapeutic indication was "replenishing the kidney *yin* and reducing the liver fire" (*ziyin pinggan* 滋阴平肝). The patient was prescribed *qiju dihuang tang* 杞菊地黄汤 (the decoction of rehmanniae with fructus lycii and chrysanthymi) with additions and subtractions.

Yuzheng (stagnation illness) as the core meaning of *qingzhi* disorder demonstrates variations from stagnation to depletion, from the disordered liver function to the disordered spleen and stomach function, and to the disordered heart and kidney function. Such variations as shown above appear in different cases, yet they also appear in the same pathological process. A patient's illness condition may go through different syndrome configurations responding to the dynamic clinical process of attuning (*tiao* 调), which will be analyzed in the next chapter.

Clinical Process of *Tiao* (Attuning)

In the previous chapters, I have discussed various cultural, sociohistorical, and ethnomedical contexts in which *qingzhi* 情志 (emotion) disorders are conceptualized, talked about, and experienced. My analysis has covered sociocultural and medical constructions of Chinese body-person, emotions, emotion-related disorders, and particularly stagnation (*yu* 郁). The present chapter, focusing on the *zhongyi* clinical process, examines how the pattern (*zheng* 证) of a particular *qingzhi* disorder case is defined through ordinary clinical work and how the process of attuning/adjusting (*tiao* 调) works to transform the patient's experience[1]. An underlying idea is that a close look at an actual face-to-face clinical communication maintained jointly by both doctor and patient can provide an important insight into the clinical construction of *qingzhi* disorders and the dynamics of *zhongyi* clinical actions and interactions. In this chapter, I deliberately incorporate techniques of microanalysis as an ethnographic tool in place of an ordinary case study that normally does not account for interactional aspects of clinical activities. I use actual recorded clinical interactions transcribed according to the conventions of conversation analysis (CA)[2], examine closely the interactive features and structures of communication between a *zhongyi* doctor and his patient, and trace how a particular syndrome pattern is determined and the path to efficacy is negotiated among the multiple clinical realities of Chinese medicine.

MICROANALYSIS AND ITS RELEVANCE TO *ZHONGYI* CLINICAL ENCOUNTERS

There has been an extensive English literature on studies of clinical communication and interactions between doctor and patient. Particularly, over the last two decades, various empirical studies have been developed for analysis of actual medical encounters.[3] One shared aspect of these studies is the meticulous examination of the actual communication between doctor and patient. Labov and Fanshel's book *Therapeutic Discourse* is an early example, which is based on a close sociolinguistic analysis of a fifteen-minute segment from a session between a patient and her psychotherapist.[4] In addition to sociolinguistic and other various forms of discourse analysis, the approach of CA has been widely used in microanalysis of actual clinical interaction. As the name itself suggests, CA is the study of "recorded, naturally occurring talk-in-interaction" with the goal to uncover "the tacit reasoning procedures and sociolinguistic competencies" that underlie the production and interpretation of such interactions.[5] My analysis in this chapter is particularly informed by the CA approach, which, more than other approaches to discourse, focuses on sequential organization of social interactions and describes the procedures through which participants themselves engage one another "to produce coherent and intelligible courses of action."[6] Since talk-in-interaction is also recognized as embodied social practice, CA has been appropriated to investigate the visual as well as the vocal elements of medical interactions.[7]

Conversation analysis (CA) has been widely applied in close analysis of talk in institutional settings including clinical interactions.[8] CA treats talk as sequentially organized social activities and pays ultimate attention to interactional meanings. From this perspective, conversation is organized and managed locally—utterance by utterance—in an orderly manner. The meaning of an utterance is not attributable to "what is really meant" by its speaker in terms of his/her intention or motivation, but can be uncovered from the perspective of how the participants display for one another their understanding of what is going on in their response to a previous utterance. This turn-by-turn unfolding of interaction then provides resources for the researcher to investigate what has been accomplished through the mundane face-to-face interaction. Consequently, for an analyst, meaning is fundamentally negotiated, contextualized, and contingent to the specific interactional history. This chapter takes CA's interpretive stance toward meaning in general and examines closely the interactive features and structures of communication between a senior male *zhongyi* doctor and his patient in a case of stagnation of emotions.

A typical conversation analysis of clinical interaction systematically examines the "interaction between doctors and patients as a topic in its own right."[9] The purpose of CA in such investigations is "to determine general rules governing the behavior of speakers that result in the apparent orderliness and structure of the interview."[10] This is certainly not my goal as an ethnographer. I do not attempt to discover general rules that account for the orderliness of doctor-patient interactions in *zhongyi* clinics. Rather, my intention is to do ethnography of the *zhongyi* clinical process in dealing with a particular case of *qingzhi* disorder. It is best described as a microanalytically oriented case study. The objective is to uncover what was practically accomplished through the joint effort of face-to-face interaction between the doctor and his patient. Different from more conventional ethnographic writing on Chinese medicine, the CA-informed ethnography uses the transcribed tape recordings of naturally occurring interactions situated in an ordinary unfolding of *zhongyi* clinic process as data. Using face-to-face interaction "as a strategic site"[11] for the analysis of *zhongyi* clinical encounters, this approach provides a mechanism to trace and demonstrate how and at what point various clinical decisions were made and therapeutic transformations were marked, expressed, and acknowledged. In addition, by focusing on how the participants themselves make sense of and respond to one another, such analysis helps reveal the tacit orientation of the speakers to the shared cultural norms and institutional expectations. Finally, microanalysis can be a process of discovery. As demonstrated by Jack Bilmes in his microanalysis of the mediator's role in a northern Thai negotiation, a close analysis of speech as a tool of ethnography "can bring us into most intimate contact with our data and give us insights of a sort that we cannot achieve with traditional methods."[12]

The zhongyi clinical process appears in various forms, and each actual event of doctor-patient interaction is situated in a particular context involving different participants. My intention is not to give a general account of *zhongyi* clinical interaction, nor to offer a standard description on how a *qingzhi* disorder is differentiated and handled in a *zhongyi* clinic. What is developed here is rather an analysis of a particular case with all its interactional details. The focus is not very much on discovering what most *zhongyi* doctors would do when facing similar problems, but rather on how a particular doctor and patient actually evoke the professional knowledge and experience, institutional competencies, and cultural and commonsensical logic in the course of interaction to make sense of one another and to negotiate meanings and actions. Moreover, this sequential unfolding of a particular process is also being recognized as a normal and ordinary *zhongyi* practice. In other words, *zhongyi* concepts and theories, such as *bianzheng lunzhi* (pattern differentiation and therapy determination), are approached not as a set of well-defined principles represented in the texts and explained by the scholar-physicians, but are examined based on how they are actually and differentially oriented to in a real-time clinical action and interaction. The CA-informed microanalytical approach is ultimately a meaning-centered interpretive enterprise. The sequential unfolding of the interaction is also an interpretive resource for the analyst to make sense of what is accomplished by the interactional moves. My underlying assumption is that it is in these everyday social interactions that embodied cultural values and social norms are presupposed, evoked, transacted, and reinforced and that cultural traditions are transmitted.

On preparing for this chapter, I listened repeatedly to the clinical encounters that I taped during my fieldwork. As I listened to exchanges among doctors, patients, family members, and myself the anthropologist, as well as other sounds of activities in the clinic—coughs, the banging of doors, the moving of chairs—the scenes of the clinical activities once more became alive to me, as if I was transferred back to the clinic. Yet any form of transcription of a naturally occurring interactional event into a written text is a form of rendering. Although I use various signs and markers to indicate intonation, pause, prolonged pronunciation, repetitions, overlaps or false starts, the distance between an actual event and a transcribed text is inevitable. My analysis relies very much on my field experience and my sense of the place, as well as years of research on Chinese medicine. I use transcripts as tools to help me "see" interaction clearly and to enable "readers to 'see' what is being referred to in analysis."[13] For this latter purpose, I also make the doctor and patient speak English. The English translation of the transcription is a rendering of a rendering, my interpretation of what is communicated between the doctor and the patient.

A face-to-face interaction involves coordination of more than just speech. I do believe that for clinical interaction, video-recorded interactions may do a better job. However, in the situation of my fieldwork, video recording was too intrusive to be of practical use. Therefore, readers have to depend on my descriptions of what was visually going on in the clinic. Frequently, silence is not real silence in terms of no action. For instance, in the case that is analyzed in this chapter, after the patient sat down, the doctor took her medical records (*bingli* 病历 in the form of a small blue booklet) and silently pushed over a soft pad. The patient put her wrist on the pad. The doctor then started to take her pulse. With his fingers on the patient's wrist, he looked at the patient with a smile. Then the patient started to talk. On the tape, we do not hear the doctor's question. Yet, by his gaze, smile, and his display of readiness, he communicated his inquiry "Where is your discomfort? (*nar bu shufu* 哪儿不舒服). Both doctors and patients constructively use silence. Understanding lies not only in something said but frequently in something unsaid. However, since I do not have recorded visual data to account for the silence except for my own memories and notes, I focus my microanalysis more on segments of conversation that were carried out more intensively and more tightly structured.

Microanalysis of face-to-face clinical interactions has been predominantly restricted to the English-speaking context and nonethnographic writing. This raises the issue as to what extent this approach of examining "talk" between doctor and patient is applicable in the understanding of *zhongyi* clinical work, which is often characterized as involving little talk.

A clinical encounter in China, known as "*kanbing*" (looking at illness by both doctor and patient) in both *zhongyi* and *xiyi* (Western biomedicine) contexts, is an interactional process.[14] In *zhongyi* clinics, this process is specifically understood as *tiao* (attuning, adjusting, balancing). Although not an officially defined *zhongyi* concept, *tiao* is characteristically employed by both doctor and patient to describe *zhongyi* therapeutics. For example, patients like to talk about finding a *zhongyi* doctor to help "attune" themselves a little (*zhao ge zhongyi daifu tiao yi tiao* 找个中医大夫调一调); similarly a doctor may suggest that a patient take some herbal medicine to regain her balance (*chi dianr zhongyao tiao yi tiao* 吃点儿中药调一调). The use of *tiao* implies that *zhongyi* therapy is a gradual and carefully managed process. It involves differentiation of a group of physical, emotional, and social dysfunctions and flexible use of available techniques, both medical and nonmedical, to "bring about the conditions" in which desirable changes in human experience and relationship can take place spontaneously.[15]

Differentiation of a particular pattern is not arrived at simply within the doctor's head, and it does not always work according to textbook logic. A pattern differentiation emerges through the process of interactions between a particular doctor and his/her patient and as a result of negotiations between multiple perspectives and different experiences. During the clinical process of "pattern differentiation and therapy determination" (*bianzheng lunzhi* 辨证论治), a *zhongyi* doctor depends on "four examinations" (*sizhen* 四诊):" (1) gazing (*wang* 望), (2) listening/smelling (*wén* 闻), (3) questioning (*wèn* 问), and (4) feeling pulse (*qie* 切) to gather information, identify symptoms, and differentiate patterns of syndromes. Theoretically, only the *wèn* (questioning) examination involves talking; the other three examinations can be done in complete silence. However, the four examinations are not separate procedures. They overlap to form a coherent process of *kanbing*, which is a face-to-face interactive phenomenon. Very often, while the doctor is asking questions, he is also taking the pulse or observing the patient. He may recheck the patient's pulse while talking to the patient. Thus, *wèn* (questioning), as a procedure to gather information and a way to engage a patient, continues through the whole clinical process. A *zhongyi* textbook particularly points out the myth of the popular image that a really good doctor needs only to read a patient's pulse to come to a full diagnosis.[16] An experienced doctor may be quick at making connections between observed signs, or he/she may be more skillful in engaging patients without posing as an interviewer.

How much the verbal exchange weighs in a clinical encounter varies according to the situation. With some cases, doctor-patient talk may be minimal. In other cases, the doctor and patient may engage in lengthy discussions. In standard *zhongyi* textbooks, doctors are encouraged to use appropriate language to clear out (*shudao* 疏导 literally "dredge") blockages in emotion and thinking and to give suggestions (*anshi* 暗示) in order to accomplish the purpose of treatment.[17] This approach is particularly emphasized in the case of *qingzhi* disorders. With a patient suffering a *qingzhi* disorder, a doctor tends to spend more time talking to the patient, and such a patient also tends to present more social and emotional problems and ask more questions. In a case of a *qingzhi* disorder, many symptoms cannot be directly observed. For example, in one patient's medical file, the symptoms that the doctor wrote down included "vexation of heart," "feeling wronged and having tendency to weep," "lack of interest," "palpitation and short breath," "tongue pale," "coating thin and yellowish," "pulse strung" and so on. It is notable that, except for the symptoms related to the tongue and pulse, all the other symptoms, particularly those about emotions, came from the patient's self-report.

Although a senior *zhongyi* doctor is respected for his or her clinical experience, as noted by Judith Farquhar, patients in a *zhongyi* clinic seldom submit themselves completely to the authority of the doctor. They also actively engage the doctor in their perspectives, help define their own illness, and even negotiate their own treatment.[18] To see the clinical encounter only as a mode of action in which the doctor masterfully deploys knowledge and resources to effect a cure is to miss a basic fact of *kanbing*. The determination of whether a certain complaint is an illness, what illness it is, what therapeutic strategy should be adopted, and what formula should be used are very much interactively interpretive and negotiated matters contingent to the clinical moment. In addition, the doctor-patient relationship in a *zhongyi* clinic is generally less structured, as both doctor and patient initiate topics and bring in their own personal experience. For a patient, this may not seem unique since a patient is expected to talk about his/her illness experience.

THE CASE OF STAGNATION OF EMOTIONS

The microanalysis of a clinical encounter in this chapter is based on a case of stagnation of emotions. The patient was a female middle-school teacher in her late twenties. She first came to the clinic in June 1994. She had been to a psychiatric hospital for her insomnia and had been prescribed some form of tranquilizers. When she came to the *zhongyi* clinic, she was still taking biomedicine but was anxious to get rid of the drug completely. Based on my observation, patients try different ways to treat their illnesses, using both biomedicine and *zhongyi*. A common explanation they give is that they seek biomedical help for immediate relief of symptoms but come to *zhongyi* for a slower process of *tiao* to redress the root(s) of their problems. This does lend some credence to the popular belief that Western medicine treats immediate symptoms (*xiyi zhibiao* 西医治标) and Chinese medicine treats the root of the problem (*zhongyi zhiben* 中医治本).

Like a typical patient with a *qingzhi* disorder, the patient complained about her distressed "heart," such as "vexed heart-emotions" (*xinqing fanzao* 心情烦躁), "uneasy feeling in the heart" (*xinli bu tashi* 心里不塌实), and "the feeling of blockage in the heart" (*xinli du de ganjue* 心里堵的感觉), as well as the physical discomforts of feeling pressure in the chest and numbness in the head. She had been divorced for two years. Although she insisted that the divorce itself was not a big trauma for her, and that she felt it was a relief, she felt her heart-emotion not flowing smoothly (*xinqing bu shuchang* 心情不舒畅) since she had not satisfactorily resolved her "personal problem" (meaning not being able to find someone to date or marry) in the ensuing two years.

In my conversation with her, I also found that she, together with her two-year-old son, lived with her father. Sometimes her father helped her to take care of her son. She did not go into detail about this part of her life, nor did the doctor ask any detailed questions about her personal life, such as her relationship with her father and mother, her childhood, and so on. Such information is not perceived as intrinsically important in *zhongyi* clinical practice. What the *zhongyi* doctor looks for are the general effects and impacts of the particular social conditions in the patient's life that may contribute to and account for various emotional and physical difficulties. The doctor is more interested in things like financial loss, an unsatisfactory job experience, stress in the workplace and in school, problems in interpersonal relationships at work or within the family, divorce, and other changes in life. At the same time, a *zhongyi* doctor tries to redress or redirect these effects and impacts.

The patient talked more about her problems at work. She was disinclined to teach the subject that she had been trained to teach in college. She found the work of homeroom teacher (*ban zhuren* 班主任), very stressful. She told her school principal that she did not want to continue teaching, preferring to do administrative work the following semester. However, the school principal was not happy about her asking for a change in her work assignment. As a result, the patient had not been assigned any work for the following semester. The suspension frustrated her. She summarized that both her work and her personal life were not going smoothly as her heart desired (*shunxin* 顺心).

The patient's unhappy personal and social life was accompanied by various physical discomforts such as dry and bitter mouth, numbness of the scalp, pressure in the head, weakness in her shoulders and arms, and sometimes stomach discomfort. The doctor did not specifically use the term *yuzheng* (stagnation syndrome) to label the illness, but it was implied in the process of differentiation of syndromes and in the therapeutic principle and the herbal formulas the doctor designed for the patient. For the first visit, the therapeutic principle was to dredge the liver system, reorder the circulation of *qi* (*shugan liqi* 疏肝理气) dissolve the stagnation, and eliminate vexation (*jieyu chufan* 解郁除烦). The patient was given the ready-made Tea of Dissolving the Stagnation and Calming the Mind (*jieyu anshen chongji* 解郁除烦冲剂) and a prescription of herbal medicine of modified decoction of Bupleuri for dispersing the depressed liver *qi* (*chaihu shugan san* 柴胡疏肝散).

One week later, the patient came back for a second visit. She looked brighter and claimed that her health had improved. She felt less vexed. However, her other symptoms, such as palpitation (*xinhuangh* 心慌), feeling of pressure in the chest (*xiongmen* 胸闷), and dry and bitter mouth (*zui gan kou ku* 嘴干口苦) were persistent. Her sleep was disturbed, too. In addition, she complained about being easily scared and jumpy (*danxiao* 胆小). She mentioned that she felt nervous and restless when she was talking to an old lady who, while talking, was constantly flapping a fan. She felt her heart was beating fast and that she had an urge to stop talking and run away, though she understood clearly there was no reason to be feeling that way. Examination found her pulse "thin and fast" and the coating of her tongue yellow. The doctor concluded the syndrome of liver *qi* stagnation had already transformed into "fire," which caused phlegm congestion. The previous prescription was modified, and new elements were added to target the recent illness development. Powdered *chengxiang* (*Chenxiang mo* 沉香末) was added to bring down the *qi* and dissolve the phlegm (*jiangqi huatan* 降气化痰). The doctor also suggested that the patient take some ready-made herbal medicine for her woman's (*fuke* 妇科) problems. He explained that in the patient's case the "wet heat" might have moved downward and caused excessive or yellowish vaginal discharge. To this the patient confirmed that she did have such symptoms.

On her third visit, the patient claimed that she felt much better. After the two previous sessions, the patient seemed to be more conformable and relaxed with the doctor. Her *xinqing* (heart-emotion) had improved; she felt less *yayi* 压抑 (depressed), and her head was not as tight and numb as before. Yet, she was anxious to know if she could completely dispense with the biomedicine that she had been using, but somehow worried that her condition would relapse if she suddenly discontinued using it. The doctor assured her that gradually she could reduce her dose of biomedicine, but there was a process, and she should be patient. From the symptoms collected and pattern differentiation shown, the doctor concluded that the patient's syndrome configuration moved from a pure repletion type to a combination type, meaning that the patient still retained some of the heteropathic factors (*xieshi*) in her system and at the same time the vital *qi* had been consumed and depleted. The therapy was designed to attack *xieshi* and also to replenish *qi* (*gongbu jianshi* 攻补兼施). The principle was to replenish *qi*, nourish the blood (*yiqi yangxue* 养气补血), further dissolve stagnation, and eliminate vexation. The patient did not come back to the clinic after the third visit.

The whole process can be easily identified as three stages. At the first stage, the symptom configuration was summarized as *yu* (stagnation), and the therapy was designed to dissolve the stagnation by activating circulation of *qi*. At the second stage, the syndrome configuration changed and was summarized as *huo* (fire), and the therapy was changed accordingly to clear fire. At the last stage, the syndrome type was identified as having *xu* (depletion) elements, and the therapeutic decision was made to incorporate replenishing measures. I was present at all three of her visits and was able to tape record the first and the last of her clinical visits. The analysis in this chapter is based mainly on the clinical interaction recorded in the patient's first visit.

DIAGNOSING YU (STAGNATION OF EMOTIONS)

The clinical process of *tiao* starts with the differentiation of syndrome pattern among an array of physical, emotional, and social dysfunctions and difficulties. There are many possible ways that symptom manifestations can be grouped and differentiated in practice. *Zhongyi* classification seeks to summarize or characterize an illness condition at a particular moment, and it certainly opens up to a range of possible interpretations that are influenced by a particular doctor's strength, training, and styles. Some doctors are good at using various replenishing methods, and others may tend to use methods of activating blood and dissolving coagulation very often. Physicians may also emphasize different visceral systems. Dealing with the same illness manifestations, one doctor may choose to start with "harmonize the stomach system" (*hewei* 和胃), and another may choose to "eliminate liver heat" (*qing ganre* 清肝热). Sometimes the same doctor may arrive at more than one characterization of a syndrome configuration and have several possible therapeutic methods prepared. If one therapy fails, he will switch to another formula.

However, it is in the interactional process of "looking at illness" that all these different factors and possibilities are played out. In the patient's illness record booklet, in the entry for the first visit, the doctor wrote down the differentiated syndrome pattern as *ganqi yujie* (liver *qi* stagnation) induced by "emotion-mind not flowing freely and smoothly" (*ingzhi bushu* 情志不舒) "the liver system losing its ability to stretch and extend" (*an shi tiaoda* 肝失条达), and the therapeutic principle of "dredging the liver and reordering the flowing of *qi*" (*shugan liqi*) and "dissolving stagnation and eliminating vexation" (*jieyu chufan*). Anyone with a little *zhongyi* knowledge can recognize that the case is diagnosed and treated as a particular *qingzhi* disorder, *yuzheng* (stagnation illness). In the transcript, the most obvious revelation of this differentiation of pattern comes from turn 68 (See transcript segment 7.4),[19] in which the doctor says: "Let's do dissolving stagnation and eliminating vexation. [Her case is that] heart-emotion is quite depressed." One interesting question then is how the doctor comes to this specific revelation at this particular point in the conversation. If we accept that differentiation of patterns is also an interactional process, then through an examination of interactional exchanges between the doctor and patient, we should be able to discover the interactional history leading to this specific diagnosis and to trace how this particular diagnosis emerged from a process of dynamic interaction between the doctor and the patient.

The patient starts her report without waiting for the doctor to question her. From the transcript (see transcript segment 7.1),[20] we can see her first turn covers a range of symptoms including both emotion-oriented complaints and somatic symptoms. Heart-emotion vexed and uneasiness in heart seem more psychological, while heart flustering and tightness and numbness of the scalp are more obviously somatic. In turn 2, the doctor simply responds to the patient's multiple complaints by repeating a single symptom, "vexation," using a more medically significant term *xinfan* than *xinqing lao fanzao* (心情老烦躁), a term used by the patient. Apparently, what the doctor is doing here is reformulating the patient's illness experience into a more medically relevant symptom (*zheng* 症). It is noticeable that out of the several complaints, only *xinfan* is immediately mentioned, but not any other symptoms. A *zhongyi* doctor routinely jots down the symptoms that are most interesting to him while listening to the patient's narrative of illness. The doctor might just simply vocalize what he is writing down in the patient's illness record booklet. But the sequential place of the utterance makes it an official response to the previous turn, which is understood and addressed by the patient as such in the next turn. Interactively, turn 2 may have several possible interpretations. It can be a question directed to the patient for confirmation. It can also be an acknowledgement the doctor offers to show that he is following the patient's report. And it may be both. Turn 3 shows that the patient is oriented to the sequential organization and reads the doctor's utterance as asking for confirmation. In the first three turns, *xinfan* becomes the most conspicuous symptomatic component of the illness.

Heart flusters (*xinhuang* 心慌), a somatic complaint, is not mentioned again in the whole interview. If the doctor in the second turn picks up *xinhuang* instead of *xinfan*, the whole interactive course may be different. At least, the fourth turn, "feeling wronged," would not be there. Instead, the most logical symptoms to look for would be "shortness of breath" (*qiduan* 气短) or "tiredness or fatigue" (*fali* 乏力), or other related somatic symptoms. If confirmed, the pattern will point to a possible configuration of a depleted pattern rather than a stagnation pattern as this case is defined. So, in a sense, the second turn shows a doctor's personal judgment where his personal experience (*jingyan* 经验) is displayed. In this case, he unambiguously directed his attention to the emotional aspect, rather than a somatic one, of the patient's suffering at the very early stage of the clinical interaction. It is also noticeable that *xinfan* is the first symptom that the patient reports. To an experienced doctor, this initial position adds importance to that particular symptom. However, the patient in discussion shows she is also "experienced" and perceptive in regards to her own illness, and her illness narrative is consistently oriented to "heart-emotion" vexation.

Experienced clinicians look for the relationships of symptoms to each other. Individual symptoms by themselves mean little. It is the symptoms appearing together that enable one pattern to be differentiated from another. *Xinfan* by itself does not tell much about what syndrome pattern the patient is suffering. What matters is with what group of symptoms it appears. In a way, at least to an experienced doctor, it suggests where to look. When an experienced doctor sees one symptom, he makes the connection to other symptoms. So in turns 4 and 6, the doctor asks if the patient feels wronged and frustrated (*weiqu* 委屈). The doctor is looking for an association of symptoms to discover an underlying pattern. The doctor's inquiry received a strong confirmation from the patient in turn 7.

Turn 8 "anxious" (*jiaolu* 焦虑)" is not articulated in a clear question form and seems ambiguous.[20] But since we understand that the doctor is looking for patterns of symptoms, the utterance could be reasonably seen as a guess, subject to confirmation or denial. In contrast to turn 7, the first part of the patient's turn 9 gives an ambiguous noncommittal "*uhn*" and then proceeds to a new information sequence by "*ranhou*" (and).[21] Analysis of the utterance of "*uhn*" is significant for understanding turn 8 and the following conversational development.

Examining closely the sequential organization, turns 8 and 9 are clearly produced as an adjacency pair in that when 8 is produced, 9 becomes conditionally relevant to 8. The utterance of "*uhn*" is indeed produced and apparently accepted as a response to 8. As I listened repeatedly to this part of the conversation, I was puzzled by this utterance of "*uhn*." If 8 is a question produced for

Transcript Segment 7.1

1.	P: a:*mm (.5) jiùshì xīnqīng lǎo fánzào: mm: ránhòu (. . .) xī:nhuā: ng (. .) jiùshi (. . .) nèige xīnl gǎnjué bù tāshi (.) jiùshi (. . .) nǎoguā pí zhèidiǎnr fǎj n (. .) fǎmá: de gǎnjué (.) ah:: (.5) jiù zhèdiǎnr (.) hòumian zhèr*	1.	P: Umm: (.5) Just that my heart-emotion has been feeling vexed. Mm: And (. .) my heart feels flustered (. .), and I've been feeling **uneasy** in my heart. And, the skin of my head feels tight and (. .) numb (.) ah:: (.5) It is right here (.) back here.
2.	D: *xīnfán*	2.	D: Heart vexed.
3.	P: *àh: xīnfán: (.)//ránhòu:=*	3.	P: Yeah:: heart vexed (.) //an:d =
4.	D: *//ěiqu me*	4.	D: //Feeling wronged?
5.	P: *=áh:*	5.	P: =wha:t?
6.	D: *w iqū: ma:*	6.	D: Feeling wronged?
7.	P: ***wěiqū:: jiù** xiǎng kū::he::hh:* ((laugh))	7.	P: **Yes:: just** feel like crying he::hh: ((laugh))
8.	D: *jiāol*	8.	D: Feeling anxious.
9.	P: *ahn (.5) ránhòu ehm:::jiùshi: ehm: (.5) z nme shuō ne (.) duì shénme shì ba: (. .) ehm hǎoxiang*	9.	P: Uhn (.5) and then uhm::: tha:t um:(.5) how can I say (.) for anything: (. .) um seems
10.	D: *=méi shénme xìngqu*	10.	D: =Do not have that much interest
11.	P: *=bù gǎn shénme xìngqu:bù gǎn shénme xìngqu:*	11.	P: =Not that interested: not that intere:sted.
12.	D: *y umeiy u shénme búliáng cìji (.) y umeiy u ah: zuìjìn*	12.	D: Have you been through any trauma (.) Have you ah: recently?
13.	P: *ahmm:*	13.	P: Uhm::
14.	D: *huòshi shēnghuó shang (.) y umeiy u shénme bù yúkuài de shìqing (.) shēnghuó shang y umeiy u āh:*	14.	D: Or in your everyday life (.) are there any unhappy things happening (.) in your everyday life are there any:?

eliciting information, 9 should be an answer. However, "*uhn*" is too vague to be a real answer. In addition, there is no reason for the patient not to give a clear yes or no answer. If the patient has no problem talking about vexation, feeling wronged, and weeping, she should have no reason to be vague about feeling anxious. However, there is no reason for the patient to hesitate in giving a negative answer to a question eliciting symptomatic information. In fact, patients understand the importance of giving accurate information. Then, why is "*uhn*" there? The logical inference is that the patient does not read the doctor's utterance in 8 as a simple question.

The doctor's utterance 8 is similar in form to turn 2. As is mentioned, 2 demonstrates the doctor's judgment as an experienced clinician. The 8 does a similar thing. By simply saying *jiaolu*, the doctor is claiming that the patient is experiencing the symptom of "*jiaolu*." The symptoms to which the doctor pays attention, such as *xinfan* (vexation), *weiqu* (feeling wronged/sad), and *jiaolu* (anxiety/nervousness) all have a "psychological" implication and are recognized by experienced doctors as symptoms that possibly go together. My *zhongyi* teacher liked to say that a good doctor, when seeing one phenomenon, is able to trace it to a different but related phenomenon. So in a way, a doctor tends to display her virtuosity of healing by making informed and intelligent guesses about what a patient may be experiencing while moving along with clinical examinations. This clinical element has always been important in *zhongyi* practice. This is where the popular belief comes from that a really great doctor can grasp the whole condition of illness just by looking at a patient or taking the pulse. There have been many legendary stories about physicians who identify illnesses and their intensity by just observation and pulse taking.[22] In the case under discussion, with the symptoms of *xinfan* and *weiqu* confirmed, *jiaolu* is very likely to coexist. The doctor in 8 is making an informed guess and displaying his knowledge and experience.

Then, a reply to 8 in a social sense is a comment on the doctor's effectiveness and virtuosity. In terms of conversational structure, turn 8 is a claim about another participant's experience, which inevitably makes the next turn relevant to the claim as either a confirmation or a denial. Any answer is consequential in both a social and a conversational sense. Then, the patient's ambiguous "*uhn*" begins to make sense.

From turn 9, we see that the patient is very reluctant to reject the doctor's claim directly but at the same time does not feel strongly enough to admit it. Considering that both the doctor and the patient have been into the interview for just a few minutes, a direct rejection to the doctor's claim, which has a special social implication in the *zhongyi* context, would be somewhat abrupt to a much-desired, smooth clinical interaction. Yet, to the doctor, the conversation participant, 9 may be indirect but not terribly ambiguous. According to the concept of "preference" in conversation analysis, not all the possible second part to a first part of an adjacency pair is of equal standing. Responses to a certain first action or part are organized by a preference system. According to Bilmes:

> Preference operates with three (or more) alternatives: a preferred (X), a non-preferred (Y), and no mention of X or Y (N). The principle is simply that, if X is preferred, N implies Y. It is this principle that, in all cases, defines preference.[23]

In the case of 8 and 9, we may say that after a claim, a confirmation is preferred. If no clear confirmation or denial takes place, it is confirmation that is officially absent, and a denial is therefore implied. The doctor must have interpreted the meaning of the first part of 9 as a denial to his claim. After "uhn" there is a short pause that could be a potential transitional point for the next turn. But unlike what he did with his previous turns (4 and 8) after the confirmation, the doctor does not take his turn at the immediate transitional point. Given the doctor's interactional pattern shown in the previous turns, if, in any case, the doctor reads the "uhn" as a confirmation, he would probably continue tracing the symptoms that are likely to go together with *jiaolu* such as "restless" (*zuowo buan* 坐卧不安)," "insomnia" (*shimian* 失眠), and so on. These symptoms if occurring with certain tongue and pulse diagnosis may suggest a syndrome configuration of depletion or an illness of visceral agitation (*zangzao* 脏躁). Yet, from turn 9 the conversational course seems to steer away from that line of inquiry.

Turn 9 does two things: it responds to 8 and introduces new information. With many pauses and hesitations, as well as a presequence "how can I say," the patient is trying to formulate an apparently not quite comfortable statement about her own experience. Anticipating what the patient is likely to say, the doctor in turn 10 says, "not have much interest." He actually completes the sentence for the patient. Again, turn 10 has the quality of displaying the doctor's judgment and understanding, which is then confirmed by turn 11. From the utterances of 9 to 11, the doctor and patient achieve a renewed alignment. Throughout the conversation, we see that both the doctor and patient are closely oriented to each other, engaging themselves in interpreting the previous turns, adjusting and repairing their utterances, and projecting the course of interaction.

By turn 11, it has been confirmed that the patient has experienced the symptoms of vexation, feeling wronged and sad, weeping, and lack of interest. It should be fairly clear to the doctor that the patient suffers from a *qingzhi*-related disorder. But it is still not sufficient to enable a particular pattern to be differentiated from other patterns. Since a *zhongyi* pattern of syndrome is a characterization of a specific illness condition with an array of physical, emotional, and social dysfunctions and difficulties, for an obvious *qingzhi*-related case, a doctor's examinations often includes questions about a patient's social experience. It is also the pattern of the patient's social experience that is informative to the task of pattern differentiation for a likely emotion-related disorder.

Turn 12 initiates a new direction in the conversation. By asking if the patient has experienced any trauma (*buliang ciji* 不良刺激) in her life, the doctor, on the one hand, evokes the shared ethnomedical assumption that the quality of a person's social life is also an important part of one's health by suggesting that the symptoms that have since been discussed have something to do with her social environment. On the other hand, turn 12 provides a space for the patient to talk about her social life.

Turn 13 shows that the patient is hesitating and is not quite sure how to answer the question. The doctor then reformulates his question by replacing the more technical term *buliang ciji* with ordinary language, "unhappy things" (*bu yukuai de shi* 不愉快的事). The difference between "*buliang ciji*" and "*bu yukuai de shi*" is not just that one is more technical and the other is more colloquial. The word *ciji*, meaning literally "stimulation," is not a *zhongyi* term but a popularized term of psychology. When a person is said to be "*shou ciji*" (traumatized), she or he is believed to demonstrate abnormalities as a result of quick and strong psychophysiological reactions. The expression also implies some form of weakness in personality. The patient's hesitation in 13 is not a result of her ignorance that she did not grasp the meaning of the more technical term *buliang ciji*, but as should be clear in her narrative in turn 16, it is rather a rejection to formulating her experience in terms of a passive "mechanical" reaction to an unfavorable environment. In contrast, "*bu yukuai de shiqing*" (unhappy things) is the language of everyday life, which does not entail a drastic redefinition of the patient's social experience with a negative implication of weakness. So the patient responds to the doctor's reformulated question with a strong confirmation that there have been too many unhappy things in her life.

The patient's narrative of her personal life and social situations mainly comes in three relatively long turns (see transcript segments 7.2 and 7.3). The first such turn is 17. The first unhappy thing the patient mentions is her divorce two years before. But, quickly referring back to the doctor's turn 12, she claims that the divorce was not really a "trauma" but rather a relief. The patient rejects the image of suffering from *ciji*. However, the fact that two years after she was divorced, she is still alone, is what the patient sees as an "unhappy thing" that needs to be solved. In today's China, divorce, though not something to be encouraged, is tolerable, particularly if one is able to get remarried and reintegrated into the "normal" flow of social life, so to speak. It is the concept of being single that is somewhat alien to the cultural conventions. The patient uses "*geren wenti*" 个人问题 (personal problem), which is a euphemism for "the matter of finding a spouse." In her own presentation, "the unhappy thing" is the lack of change in her personal life after her divorce. The image she uses to formulate her experience is blockage and stagnation (*butong* 不通). Because of the blockage in her social life, her heart-emotion "is always feeling blocked" (*bu shuchang*不舒畅).

On top of blockage and stagnation in her personal life, another important topic that echoes through the entire conversation is her unhappiness with her job. The patient tells the doctor that she is not just a middle school-teacher. She is a homeroom teacher (*ban zhuren* 班主任) who teaches two subjects. The repeatedly used sentence structure "*ranhou ba wo you* ... (then ... I also)" piles up one job on another, communicating feelings of pressure and stress, especially considering the shared assumption about what it is like to be an elementary or middle-school teacher in China. They are seen as having too many responsibilities, too little pay, and too much work. In a Chinese school, students in one class (*ban*), usually forty to sixty, stay together for all their classes and many extracurricular activities throughout their years in that school (in elementary school they stay together in one *ban* for six years; in middle school three years, and in high school three years). A homeroom teacher is ultimately responsible for all concerns of the *ban*—academic, social, and emotional—but he or she seldom teaches more than one subject. In turn 18, the doctor's repetition of "two subjects" in a rising tone at the end shows his surprise that the patient besides being the homeroom teacher also teaches two subjects. In a way, the utterance shows that the doctor is paying particular attention to the patient's report and is sympathetic with her situation.

After several exchanges about what subjects the patient teaches and where she graduated, the patient continues her narrative in turn 29. The continuation is clearly marked by the same sentence construction (*ranhou ba wo you* . . .). She piles on top of her job stress the stress of being a single mother. For the second time in her narration she says "My heart-emotion has been for a long time feeling blocked" (not flowing smoothly and freely). Then she characterizes her social situation by saying, "Both my personal life and work have not been going too smoothly" (not following my heart's desire). Later, in turn 57, after talking about her unhappy experience at the workplace, the patient again claims: "I feel very uncomfortable in my heart. (.5) I: feel (. .) extremely wronged and vexed." The Chinese term is *wonang* 窝囊. It is a combined feeling of being wronged without a channel to vent the frustration and heart-emotion not flowing freely. A consistent metaphor in the patient's narrative is "not flowing" (*bu shuchang* 不舒畅), and the image is blockage and stagnation.

In *zhongyi* clinical context, we see that illness experience recognizes no boundaries between what is social, psychological, or physical. In fact, the

---

Transcript Segment 7.2

---

15. P: *tài duō le (. .) hǎoxiàng shi::* hei: hh ((laugh))

15. P: *Too* many (. .) I suppose :: hei::hh: ((laugh))

16. D: uh: ha hh ((laugh))

16. D: uh: ha hh ((laugh))

17. P: *yīnwéi (.3) w ba: en:: jiùshi: (.5) liǎng nián qián (.5) líhūn le (3) qíshí ba:: líhūn ba:: búshì shénme cìji (.8) w juéde shì yì zh ng jiětuō ha: dànshì jiùshi:: guò yí duàn shíjiān ba:: w jué de: jiùshi:: en:: zōngshì bùnéng:: yuǎnmǎn de jiějué w de gèrén wèntí (.5) xīnl ba:: lǎoshì bù shūchàng (.) ránhou w búshì dāng jiàoshī me (.) ránhòu w yòu zuò bānzh rèn gōngzuò (.) ránhòu w yòushì:: jiāo: liǎng mén kèchéng (.3) ah::n*

17. P: Because (.3) I um:: tha:t (.5) two years ago (.5) was divorced (.3) Actually uh:: divorce was not that much a trauma (.8) I *feel* it's a kind of relief uh:: *But* that:: after some time uh:: I fe:lt that:: uh:: I *just* can not solve my personal problem satisfactorily (.5) My heart-emotion uh:: is always feeling blocked ((not flowing smoothly and freely)) (.) And then I am also a teacher. And then I am also a homeroom advisor (.) and then I also:: teach: two subjects (.5). Ah::n

18. D: *liǎng mén kèchéng*

18. D: Two different subjects?

language the patient uses to talk about her experience does not require these distinctions. For example, expressions such as "not flowing freely" (*bu shuchang*)," "blocked" (*du* 堵)," "pressed and suffocated" (*bie* 憋)," and "not smooth" (*bu shun* 不顺), are used in describing emotional, social, and physical experience. Complaints in any of these aspects are all recognized as symptomatic and contribute to an overall picture of the illness. The much talked about *zhongyi* "holism" is not a conceptual abstract but a concrete reality unfolded in *zhongyi* clinical interactions.

After the patient's utterance (29) that both her personal life and her work have not been going smoothly, the doctor's next question (31) is, "Do you have a stuffy chest?" The doctor is now ready to direct his inquiring gaze to the physical symptoms that correspond to the patient's social and emotional experience. The patient answers, "just feel like:: suffocated//difficult in drawing a breath (32)." The patient uses colloquial words for "suffocated" (*bie* 憋) and "difficult in drawing a breath" (*shangbulai qi* 上不来气). Again, the difference between the doctor's terminology and the patient's is not that the former is more technical, and the later is more colloquial. In fact, the word that the doctor uses "the stuffy chest" (*xiongmen* 胸闷) is also a common term. Since utterance 32 is not clearly indicated as a negative answer to the doctor's question, the patient must have perceived her experience as somehow similar or at least comparable to that of the symptom of "the stuffy chest." Yet, by using her own expressions, she characterizes her experience as something that does not totally conform to the doctor's characterization from an apparently medical perspective. *Xiongmen* (the stuffy chest) is a common symptom in *yuzheng* (stagnation illness). It is understood by *zhongyi* doctors as originating from a disordered *qi* circulation that causes *qi* to accumulate and to be trapped in the liver system, and the patient then experiences a feeling of fullness and pressure in the chest. *Xiongmen*, therefore, as *zhongyi* terminology, is more a medicalized description of *qi* gathered inside without an outlet, or of *qi* blocked from flowing out. However, the patient uses *bie* (suffocated) and *shangbulai qi* (difficult breathing) to describe her experience of obstructed breathing. The emphasis is more on the blockage that obstructs the vital *qi* of life from coming inside. The doctor's characterization focuses more on disordered internal mechanism that is central to the patient's illness, while the patient's description sees the external pressure (literally and figuratively) as a more significant factor.

When the doctor hears the patient say "*bie de*," he immediately cuts in and asks if the patient tends to exhale a long breath (33), because *bie* has both meanings of "suppress" and "suffocate." If the patient uses the former meaning of the term, 32 would be a fully positive answer to turn 31. The image of wanting to give out long breaths is an extension of "*xiongmen*," since if *qi* is suppressed inside the chest, the patient tends to help *qi* out by breathing out hard and long. A more technical term is giving constant sighs (*xi taixi* 喜太息)." The doctor's question in turn 33 overlaps the patient's second half of turn 32, which shows that "*bie*" is actually used in its second sense as "suffocate." Therefore, although

Transcript Segment 7.3

29. P: *Uh:: (.) ránhòu ba: w* *zìj yòu dài háizi: uh: jiùshi* *xīnqíng chángqī de lǎo::shi bù:* *shūchàng (.5) jiùshi shēnghuó* *shang: gōngzuò shang dōu:: bú* *tài shùnxīn::*	29. P: : Uh:: (.) then: I also take care of my chi: ld by myself. Uh: that my heart-emotion has been for a long: time feeling blocked and unhappy (.5) and both my personal life: and work are not going satisfactorily::
30. D: *((talk to a previous patient* *who came back to ask some* *questions about how to take the* *medicine)) (15)*	30. D: ((talk to a previous patient who came back to ask some questions about how to take the medicine)) (15)
31. D: *xiōng mèn bu mèn ah::*	31. D: Do you have a stuffy chest ah::?
32. P: *jiùshi:: biē de //shàngbulái qì*	32. P: Just:: feel like suffocated// difficult drawing a breath.
33. D: *//x huān cháng chūqì shìma:*	33. D: //Tend to give out a long breath, right?
34. P: *àh:::*	34. P: Yeh:::
35. D: *=shì zhèyang me ((the* doctor draws a deep breath and lets it out as if giving out a sigh))	35. D:= Like this? ((The doctor draws a deep breath and lets it out as if giving out a sigh.))
36. P: *àh: shàngbulái qì: (.) a:* *h: ránhòu zhè dìfang d* *de tè nánshòu::: a:h y u* *shíhou ba: jiùshi xīn l fán* *de shíhou ba:: w jiù juéde* *wèicháng gōngnéng ba: jiùshi* *hǎoxiàng::(.) y u diǎnr yòu* *xiǎng lā dùzi dànshì yòu* *méiy u*	36. P: *Yeh: have difficulty in drawing* a breath. Uh: then here feels like something stuck and **very** uncomfortable::: u:h ((the patient presses one hand on the area that Chinese usually call "the mouth of the heart")). Sometimes: when:: my heart feels vexed, I feel the function of my stomach and bowels seems to be: (.) sort of like diarrhea but actually it is not.

by utterance 34 "*uh*" the patient gives a confirmation to the doctor's turn 33, the doctor hears the patient's second half of 32 "difficult in drawing a breath" as somehow contradictory to her confirmation in 34. He quickly adds another question to follow up, this time by demonstration. He draws in a deep breath first and then lets it out slowly. Interestingly, the patient says "*uh*" to confirm the doctor's demonstration, but at the same time, insists on "*shangbulai qi*" (difficult breathing in). The feeling of blockage at any point normally does involve two-way movement: in and out. However, *zhongyi* doctors see as the central illness mechanism the stagnant *qi* stuck within one's system and thus blocking the flow of both in and out. *Zhongyi* recognizes that it is crucial to activate the person's own systems to move the stagnant *qi* first. This strategy is reflected in many *zhongyi* therapeutic methods, such as "dredging" (*shu* 疏)," "releasing" (*xie* 泄), "dispersing" (*jie* 解), and "draining" (*tong* 通). However, this particular patient focuses almost stubbornly on the difficulty of breathing in. Her repeated use of the expression *shangbushanglai qi* (can't breathe) seems to be her bodily comment on her stagnant personal life and suppressive social environment. In everyday Chinese language, people often use similar expressions, such as *chuan buguo qi lai* to describe suffocation and suppression of one's social and political environment.

Finally, the doctor gets a clearer confirmation when the patient presses her hand on her upper stomach area saying she feels uncomfortable as if there is something stuck there. This in some way supports the doctor's analysis, because according to *zhongyi* physiology and pathology the accumulated stagnant *qi* in the liver system is very likely to encroach on the stomach system and cause a feeling of fullness and pressure. In the record booklet the doctor used "feeling fullness and blockage in the chest and stomach area" (*xiongwan biemen* 胸脘 憋闷). He managed to combine both *men* (stuffy) and *bie* (suffocation) in one symptom and was able to accommodate the patient's point of view.

By now, the emotional symptoms, social difficulties, and physiological symptoms have been considered. Before turn 68, the doctor asks to look at the patient's tongue. Then the examination is completed, and the diagnosis in terms of differentiation of patterns is reached. We notice that the patient is continuing to provide information on her illness in turn 67 saying that she also feels fatigue. Apparently, the patient's 67 utterance about lack of strength is not addressed by the doctor in the following turn. In fact, the patient's complaint is not addressed by the doctor until the patient's third visit when the syndrome pattern of depletion (*xu* 虚) is diagnosed. It is always stressed in the *zhongyi* clinic that among complicated symptom configurations, a doctor should grasp the main conflict (*zhuyao maodun* 主要矛盾). By not addressing the new information, the doctor also indicates the end of the stage of *bianzheng* (differentiation of pattern) and the beginning of *lunzhi* (discussing treatment).[24] The doctor's utterance 68 begins with, "Thi::s uh: is like this (.5)" which is a presequence to the coming concluding remarks. "Let's do releasing the stagnation and dissolving vexation" shows both a differentiation of syndrome pattern and determination of a therapeutic strategy. The doctor particularly mentions the patient's suppressed (*yayi* 压抑) heart-emotion as the main problem, with which the patient agrees completely (69). Apparently, the patient's condition is diagnosed as "stagnation of emotions" (*qingzhi zhi yu* 情志之郁) originated from the difficulties and problems in her social environment.[25]

In the above analysis, I have shown how the *zhongyi* diagnostic process of differentiation of patterns (*bianzheng*) works in one particular case. I have tried to trace the origin of the diagnosis of *yu* and demonstrate how this particular pattern differentiation emerges as the result of the process of interaction and negotiation between the doctor and the patient. The purpose is not to present the standard practice of *bianzhen lunzhi* (pattern differentiation and therapy

Transcript Segment 7.4

65. P: *háiyou:: zu :: fāgān: fāk :::*	65. P: And also:: my mouth feels dry: and bitter:::.
66. D: *w kànkan shétou kànkan: (.5) tāi bóhuáng (.5)* shézh dàn:: dàn (. . .)	66. D: Let me look at your tongue. Look at: (.5) The coating is thin and yellow (.5). The color of the tongue is pale:: pale (. . .)
67. P: *y u shíhour: ba:: juéde: ba:: cóng: jiānjiāg r:: dào liǎng ge bì ba:: juéde yì diǎn::r jìnr dōu méiy u:: méi jìnr*	67. P: Sometimes uh:: feel: uh:: from:: the shoulder blades:: to my two arms:: feel no strength at a::ll, no strength.
68. D: *(zhège:: e: shì zhèyàng) (.5) ji yù chúfán ba::(tā zhè zh ng shi:) xīnqíng b jiāo yāyì*	68. D: (Thi::s uh: is like this.) (.5) Let's do releasing the stagnation: and dissolving vexation uh:: (Her case is) heart-emotion feels quite depressed.
69. P: *àhn::: xīnqíng tè::: yā:: yì:: y u shíhòur xiǎngq zhèixiē shìr:: yuè:: xiǎng yuè:: fán: (1.5) y u shíhour (.5) jiù::jiu xiǎng::n=*	69. P: **Yeh**::: heart-emotion feels **very**::: depressed. Sometimes when thinking of these thi::ngs, **the more** I think, *the more* I feel vexed. (1.5) Sometimes (.5) ju::st ju: st wa::nt=

determination), but rather to show how a particular *zhongyi* physician, who is known for his efficacy in treating *yuzheng* (stagnation illness), particularizes this "standardized" process through his personal experience, perspectives, language, and style of communication. His attentiveness to the patient's emotional and social problems as shown in the case analyzed here may well show his particular strength that contributes to his reputation with emotion-related disorders.

NEGOTIATING A PATH TO EFFICACY

Since *zhongyi* therapy is typically understood as *tiao*, a gradual and carefully managed process of adjustment, efficacy, or effectiveness (*xiao* 效) can be assessed at any given stage of a treatment. The *zhongyi* wisdom "if effective, do not change the formula/method" (*xiao bu geng fang* 效不更方) is still evoked by physicians in clinical actions, not so much as a guiding principle but rather as useful accumulated experience (*jingyan* 经验) to indicate that *xiao* is constantly assessed so that therapeutic strategies can be adjusted accordingly.[26] In this sense, *xiao* or *liaoxiao* 疗效 has the meaning of "proximate effects that indicate the healing/curing process is under way." However, *xiao* is also used to mean "the ultimate outcome" of a treatment.[27] For the purpose of this analysis, *xiao* or *liaoxiao* is glossed as both effectiveness and efficacy. I use them interchangeably with the former to indicate more "proximate effects" and the latter more "as the ultimate outcome."

In the *zhongyi* clinical encounter, the patient's own narrative on how effective or not effective a particular treatment is plays an important role in the doctor's decision to change a therapy or to retain a current one. While it is true that the *zhongyi* doctor cannot reject the patient's own presentation of the effects of a treatment, the doctor, having professional training and experience, is able to put in medical perspective the signs observed and reported by the patient and persuade the patient to see the signs as proximate medical effects that indicate that the healing process is under way. *Zhongyi* treatment emphasizes healing as a process; thus proximate effects are given considerable attention. The concept *"tiao"* (attuning or balancing) itself suggests that *zhongyi* therapy is a long-term task. Since the "ultimate efficacy" of being "attuned" or balanced cannot be absolute and timeless, *tiao* might be a lifelong effort.

In addition, *zhongyi* efficacy is also seen as emerging from the entire clinical process of *tiao* involving adjustments in all aspects of the patient's illness conditions. *Zhongyi* doctors assume that a person's emotions, thoughts, and visceral systems are interconnected in a functional way and that changes in one aspect would lead to changes in other aspects. They generally feel no need to make distinctions between efficacy produced by specific herbal contents and that from "nonspecific therapeutic sources."[28] Doctors consistently prescribe herbal medicine for the patients whose illness conditions are diagnosed as caused by excessive emotions or by social difficulties. Similarly, prescribing herbs does not necessarily negate the need for nonmedical "talk" to persuade the patient to change his or her perspectives. Rather, *zhongyi* doctors make use of all available sources, medical and nonmedical, to facilitate a positive change in the patient.

In the case analyzed in this chapter, a herbal medication was prescribed at all three of the patient's visits. Clearly, both doctor and patient expected that a particularly tailored herbal medication would work to activate *qi* movement and thus to dissolve the stagnation of emotions. In fact, the shared confidence in herbal interventions is very much the context in which the *zhongyi* "talk" takes place. The choice to focus on talk is not to deny effectiveness of herbal therapies but rather that the theoretical framework of microanalysis does not accommodate an adequate assessment of the role of herbs. More importantly, this analysis is not meant to assess efficacy of a given *zhongyi* therapy but to uncover the aspect of the clinical process of *tiao* that has escaped most ethnographic scrutiny, namely, the discursive attendance to emotions and thoughts.

Medical efficacy "might lie in the determination of who or what caused the illness and why that particular person was affected."[29] In other words, efficacy may start with diagnosis. As shown above, the case analyzed here was differentiated as "liver *qi* stagnation" (*ganqi yujie*) induced by "emotion not flowing smoothly" (*qingzhi bushu*) and "the liver system losing its ability to stretch and extend" (*gan shi tiaoda*). The therapeutic principle that the doctor chose was to "dredge the liver system and reorder the flow of *qi*" (*shugan liqi*) and "dissolve stagnation and eliminate vexation" (*jieyu chufan*). The above analysis is meant to show the interactional history leading to this specific diagnosis and to trace how this particular diagnosis emerged from a dynamic interaction between the doctor and patient. In the following, the focus of my analysis will be on how both doctor and patient actively negotiate over "the conditions" in which desired changes in the patient's experience may take place.

For *qingzhi* disorders, *tiao* is particularly understood as involving more than the adjustment of physiological process. Adjustment of one's perceptions and of one's social relations is also part of the attuning process and, in fact, one important condition leading to efficacy. A passage from a *zhongyi* textbook states:

> As pointed out in *Linzheng Zhinan Yi'an: Yuzheng,* "healing of *yuzheng* depends very much on a patient's ability to transform emotions and change perspectives."[30] That's why doctors should show concern for patients' sufferings, counsel the patients, fully motivate the positive elements in the patients, so that they can help the patients reorient themselves and encourage them to let go of their worries and to develop confidence in overcoming illnesses.... Depending solely on material medicine, the stagnation cannot be dissolved and efficacy is hard to achieve.[31]

In the case of the patient, the meaning of helping smooth (*shu*) and reorder (*li*) the flow of emotions and dissolve (*jie*) and eliminate (*chu*) the feeling of blockage in her social and emotional life is also embedded in the therapeutic strategy of "dredging the liver and reordering the flow of *qi*" and "dissolving stagnation and eliminating vexation."[32] Looking closely at the actual clinical interaction in the contemporary *zhongyi* practice, it is clear that doctors do engage in counseling patients. However, the way *zhongyi* doctors work with patients is different from the psychological counseling normally found in typical Western psychiatric clinics. Unlike a psychotherapist who tries to bring the patient into contact with his or her "true feelings or conflict" that are supposedly suppressed or denied by the patient, a *zhongyi* doctor has no interest in any unconscious "true" feelings. What is important to *zhongyi* counseling, shown in the following analysis of the clinical interaction, is to help the patient develop an adaptive attitude and perspective in order to better adjust to her social environment.

A *zhongyi* doctor does not pose him- or herself as an expert in emotions, but as a wise person who has accumulated practical wisdom through life and professional experiences.[33] The *zhongyi* doctor cannot assume an "objective" point of view on the patient's "emotional problem" as a psychotherapist does in therapeutic interaction. A *zhongyi* doctor very often forges a connection with the patient by transforming "the patient's problem" into shared human conditions and therefore makes it legitimate to offer moderate advice in forms of personal experience and reflections that one may hear from one's trusted friends or relatives. For example, when the patient in this case says that she does not want to teach PE and gives "poor health" as the reason, the doctor says in

reply that "frequent exercise is helpful," which is certainly a rejection of the reason that the patient offers. He then offers an anecdote about himself that one
winter his bicycle was stolen, so he had to get up early and walk to the hospital
every morning, and as a result, he never caught a cold that winter. In *zhongyi*
clinics, the so-called counseling is very much a negotiation between at least
two different points of view and perspectives informed by different knowledge,
experience, and interest. The success of negotiation depends largely on the type
of connections forged between the doctor and patient through actively managed turn-by-turn interactions.

After the differentiation of pattern and determination of therapeutic principle, the conversation moves on to talking about a medical prescription. In
turn 79 (see transcript segment 7.5 for 75–89), the doctor asks if it is okay for the
patient to take the herbal medicine that she needs to decoct by herself at home.
The patient replies that it is fine with her because she is not working these days,
meaning she has time to prepare herbal medicine. The doctor reads more into
the patient's reply. In turn 81, the doctor says, "Brew some herbal soup and just
get well fast." He then follows the same message in turn 83 "Get well fast, then
you can go back to work soon (.) Have to make money, right?" The turn refers
to the patient's utterance in turn 80 that the patient is not working; at the same
time "have to make money" is meant and heard to be a joke. The theme of "not
working" (*mei shangban* 没上班) in the patient's utterance 80 is only secondarily
mentioned and is furthermore presented as a facilitating condition. However,
the doctor picks up on this as a problem or a complaint. From turns 81 to 83,
he manages to turn it into a major topic of discussion in the conversation that
follows.

Responding to the doctor's humorous remark that she needs to get well fast
so that she can go to work and make money, the patient laughs and replies by
saying that her situation has almost become a vicious cycle and that the longer
she is not able to work, the more her heart-emotion feels vexed. The expression
she uses to characterize her situation is "unable to go to work" (*shangbuliao ban*
上不了班) rather than "not go to work" (*bu shangban*)." The patient tries to say
that her illness prevents her from going to work. The illness originates from her
vexed heart-emotion, which results from her unhappy personal life and the unresolved problems in her social world. To complete this "vicious cycle," inability
to work can only worsen her already strained relationship at her workplace.

At this point, the doctor then says, "Some amount of work will be helpful.
It is not good not to work." Sequentially and logically, the doctor's utterance
is a response to the patient's turn 87, saying that some amount of work will
help the patient feel better. But if we look at the exchanges from 80 through
88, turn 88, especially the criticism "It is not good not to work" can also be read
as a follow-up to 81 and 83, as a response to the patient's revelation that she is
not working. Especially, the mention of money in 88 makes it relevant to turn
81. If the utterance "It is not good not to work" was said at turn 81 instead of at
88, it would be understood as a direct criticism of the patient and would pose a

Transcript Segment 7.5

75. D: *ah:: w g i n kāi: diă: nr chōngjì zài: dài: kāi diănr tāngyào(.) néng chéng mā::*	75. D: uh:: I'll prescribe you some ready-made preparation and also prescribe some herbal medicine to decoct (.) Is that ok with you::?
76. P: *áh::*	76. P: Ah::?
77. D: *chōngjì zhuānmén zhì n zhège bìng de áh::*	77. D: The ready-made preparation is especially designed for treating the kind of illness you have. Okay?::
78. P: àh:: xí::ng	78. P: Ah:: Fi::ne .
79. D: *zài kāi (. .) áo diănr yào hăobuhăo::?*	79. D: And also prescribe (. .) boil some herbal medicine, is that oka::y?
80. P: *k :y :: xíng(.) făn:zhèng: xiànzài w yě méi shàngbān::*	80. P: That's fine. No problem. I am staying at home these days anyway.
81. D: *áo diănr yào: ba:: gănj n: hăo: déle*	81. D: Brew some he:rb soup and just get well fast.
82. P: *è:ng*	82. P. u:hn:
83. D: *hăo: le gănj n gōngzuò (.) háidĕi: zhèngqián ne*	83. D: Get well fast, then you can go back to work soon (.) Have to make money, right?
84. P: *ha::ha:: ((laugh))*	84. P: Ha::ha:: ((laugh))
85. P: *dōu èxìng xúnhuán le:: w pà w dōu chéng le (.) xiànzài*	85. P: Almost become a vicious cycle::now, I am afraid.
86. D: *néng hăo méi wèntí*	86. D: You'll be fine. No problem.
87. P: **yuè::** *shàng bù liăo bān: ba: xīnqíng* **yuè//făn::** *(.) juéde: e ::*	87. P: The **lo::nger** I am not able to wo:rk uh: the **mo:re** my heart-emotion feels ve: xed (.) //I fee:l uh::
88. D: *//shìdāng gōngzuò:: bù gōngzuò bùhăo:: bùdān qián de wèntí*	88. D: //Some amount of work:: is necessary. It is not good not to work. It is not just a matter of money.
89. P: *shìdāng gōngzuò ah:*	89. P: Some amount of work?

potential "loss of face" threat to the patient. When the critical comment in turn 88 "It is not good not to work" is uttered, it has been cushioned by a joke, and it is several turns removed from the original place where the topic is introduced. The patient's response is a repetition of the doctor's words "some amount of work" in a suspending tone that conveys confusion and serves as a request for further explanation. The disagreement is more subtle and fundamental than it seems. The patient presents her situation as "not able to go to work," something that is beyond her personal choice. However, the doctor's way of talking about the matter, such as "do some amount of work" (*shidang gongzuo*) and "not work" (*bu gongzuo*) challenges the patient's self-characterization and makes it sound as if the patient is somehow responsible for not going to work, which, according to the doctor, is a mistake. We sense the tension between these two perspectives. The patient sees her situation as things happening to her beyond her own control, yet the doctor sees that the key factors in the patient's illness and effective healing lie within the patient herself. The tension between the two perspectives runs throughout the entire conversation and shapes the patterns of the interaction. For example, when the patient says that she does not want to teach PE because of her poor health, the doctor rejects the patient's explanation by reversing her argument and claiming that physical exercise is actually good for the health. The earlier doctor and patient exchanges about the symptom of "fullness of the chest" (*xiongmen*) suggest a similar pattern of interaction: while the patient insists on a feeling of suffocation, "not able to breath in" (*shangbulai qi*), the doctor focuses on the feeling of fullness and pressure within her chest.

The doctor's emphasis on the patient's role in the course of illness development is consistent with *zhongyi*'s conceptualization of the *qingzhi* disorder and its healing. The stagnation syndrome (*yuzheng*) is understood particularly as originating in human conditions: "disappointment in getting what one seeks" (*suoqiu busui* 所求不遂), "failure to achieve one's goal" (*zhiyi buda* 志意不达), and so on. Its healing depends very much on the patient's ability to "transform emotions and changes" (*yiqing yizhi* 移情易志).[34] The famous Ming dynasty physician Zhang Jingyue, in his writings about *yuzheng*, says "a person who is ill because of emotions can only be healed by emotions: with a woman, her desire has to be fulfilled before her stagnation can be removed; with a man, he has to learn to be flexible and have broad heart-mind and superior wisdom, otherwise his illness can not be transformed."[35]

We can see that the doctor is trying to transform the patient's emotions and change her focus. The implied meaning of being disabled by her illness in the patient's utterance of 87 is not acknowledged in the doctor's next turn. Instead, the utterance in the doctor's turn 88 presupposes just the opposite; that is, the patient is able to work. In the patient's turn 89, by repeating the doctor's words and asking for further elaboration without addressing the question of ability to work, it seems as if the patient tacitly accepts the doctor's presupposition of utterance 88 that her "not working" is the result of her own choice rather than caused by her disability. At least, from the doctor's response in turn 90 (see transcript segment 7.6 for 90–93), we know that the doctor hears the patient's turn 89 as asking why she should work rather than if she is able to work. In turn 90, the doctor starts to explain why it is important to work, thus opening his lengthy speech to persuade (*kaidao* 开导, literally "open" and "guide," meaning to help a person see his/her situation clearly and sensibly) the patient.

The doctor in turn 90 starts with a general claim: "Human beings are like this (..) need to have a source of satisfaction (..)." Generally, a *zhongyi* doctor tries to avoid getting into the details of a patient's personal life, partly because a *zhongyi* doctor does not have the professional claim that a psychotherapist has for an authoritative voice over interpreting the patient's behavior and emotional experience. What the *zhongyi* doctor relies on is some form of relatedness between him and his patient that allows him to draw from his own experience to bear on the patient's experience, that is, the shared human condition. In addition, the practical purpose of this type of *kaidao* is to help a patient tune into a different perspective so that she can become better adjusted to her environment.

Transcript Segment 7.6

90. D: *rén jiù zhèiyà::ng (..) yào y u ge jìtuō (..) w xiǎ:ng shì zhèyang (.) h nduō lǎonián rén tuìxiū:: (.) wèishénme tā líxiū jiù róngyì dé bìng ah: bùdān shì ge qián de wèntí yīnggāi háiy u ge gōngzuò jìtuō (.) shēnghuó jìtuō wèntí (2.0)//rénde*

91. P: *//k w xiànzài shēnghuó shang gōngzuò shang yì diǎnr jìtuō dōu méiy u (..) xīnl lǎo=*

92. D: *=bù (1.0) rén y u yì zh ng (..) búshì méiy u jìtuō (.) y y u jìtuō (..) jiùshì zài n zhèr mùqián bú tài l xiǎng (...) rúgu rén sīxiǎng shang shēnghuó shang méi:y u jìtuō yì tiān y huó bú xiàqù (.) w rènwéi ta yì tiān y huó bú xiàqu (...) bāokuò zìshā de rén (.) w juéde zìshā de rén y :: h n:: ye h n: y dào yídìng de chéngdù búshì shuō:: hei:: h:: ((laugh)) juéxīn h n dà ha:: ha:: ((laugh)) (...) yìbān rén bù xíng de (.5) jiù sh:: jiù:n xiànzài búshi méi jìtuō(..) jiù: shr shuō bù l xiǎng (...) jiùshr bù hé xīn::si.*

93. P: *duì méicuòr*

90. D: Human being is like this (..) needs to have a source of satisfaction (..) I thi:nk this is true (.) Many old people when reti::red (.) why is that he tends to fall ill after retirement ah:? It is not just money: There should also be something to do with having a source of satisfaction from work (.) and life. (2.0)//A person's

91. P: //But now I do not have any source of satisfaction at all from both my work and my life (..) In my heart I always=

92. D: =No! (1.) Human being has a ki:nd (..) It is not that you do not have a source of satisfaction (.) You too have a source of satisfaction (..) Just that your present situation is not that ideal (...) If a person cannot find any satisfaction in his mind or life, he cannot live on for a single day (.) I think he is not able to live on for one day (...) including those who seek suicide (.) I think a suicidal person also:: ve::ry also ve:ry must have come to a certain degree. It is not to say:: hei:: h:: ((laugh)) must be very determined ha::ha:: ((laugh)) (...) An ordinary person is not able to do it (.5) As for:: as: your present situation, it is not that you do not have a source of satisfaction (..), it's just that it is not ideal (...), not what your heart-mind wants it to be.

93. P: **Right**. Exa::ctly.

After the doctor frames the subject as a shared human condition, he goes on to say, "I think this is true." Phrases with "I think" or "I feel" are frequently used by the doctor in his talk with the patient. The use of such expressions makes the doctor's speech less inviting of the patient's rejection or resistance. At least, the doctor is entitled to have his own point of view. Also, the status of *lao zhongyi* (senior, experienced *zhongyi* doctor) lends credibility to his words and experience. The doctor uses the example of retired people to support his claim that work is necessary (see turn 90). After he finishes the sentence that working has something to do with finding satisfaction in life, there is a long pause, indicating that the doctor expects the patient to respond and to acknowledge the importance of work other than for economic reasons. After about two seconds, seeing that the patient has made no move to respond, the doctor is obliged to continue. The patient's delayed response overlaps with the doctor's effort to continue his *kaidao*. The patient's response comes as a surprise to the doctor.

Instead of following the logic set forth by the doctor to acknowledge that continuing to work is helpful because it gives a person a sense of satisfaction in life, the patient claims, "But now I do not have any source of satisfaction at all in both my work and my life" (91). The patient's claim is quickly and forcefully rejected by the doctor, who cuts the patient's utterance short. It is noticeable throughout the transcript that the doctor is particularly sensitive to any potential assertion of negative feelings, especially feelings of hopelessness the patient may make, and does not hesitate to intervene whenever he sees one coming. For example, in turn 69, the patient claims that her "heart-emotion" is feeling low and heavy (*yayi*), and when she says, "sometimes (.5) ju::st ju::st want::, " the doctor cuts in, and the patient's sentence is not finished. From the context, the doctor sensed the unfinished utterance might be negative. Again in turn 87, the patient claims that the longer she is not able to go to work, the more vexed she feels. When she is about to continue talking about her vexed feelings, her sentence "I fee:l uh::" is interrupted by the doctor's speech. Similarly, in turn 91 the patient says that she does not have any satisfaction in work or life, and her sentence "In my heart I always" is interrupted by the doctor's forceful "No." Unlike a Western psychotherapist who frequently encourages the client to talk about emotions and particularly her negative feelings, a *zhongyi* doctor discourages the patient from talking about negative feelings and therefore refuses to make it a topic. In a *zhongyi* context it is almost seen as therapeutically healthy not to focus on negative elements of a person's experience.

In turn 92, after a quick rejection and a relatively long pause, the doctor starts to do the same thing as he did in turn 90, that is, to formulate the problem as a shared human condition. Somehow, he feels compelled to address the patient's negative evaluation of her own situation and to offset the negative overtone of the utterance by stating his rejection again. He begins with "It is not that you do not have a source of satisfaction," then there is a short pause, a would-be transitional point, but the patient does not take the turn. Then the doctor continues to contradict the patient's negative opinion and says, "You too have a source of satisfaction." This utterance is followed by another short pause that is a little longer than the previous one. The doctor's invitation for the patient to respond fails again. He then adds a more compromising comment, "Just that your present situation is not that ideal." After this utterance, there is an even longer pause. However, the doctor still fails to get the patient's response. Considering that the doctor is talking about the patient's experience and contradicting the patient's statement, the patient's lack of response implies that she insists on her own opinion and rejects the doctor's characterization of her situation. The doctor simply cannot keep talking about the patient's experience without the patient's acknowledgement in some form. He then resorts to his old strategy to make a more generalized reasoning that if a person does not have any satisfaction in life, she cannot live on for one day. As the realm has now been switched to general human behavior, the doctor gains legitimacy to give his opinions. He brings out the topic of suicide to support his case that one cannot live without any source of satisfaction in life, but he quickly discovered that this is a mistake. He is obviously uncomfortable discussing the topic in this situation. The argument about suicide is incoherent and marked by embarrassed laughs. However, after the doctor has made the point about "satisfaction in life," he returns to the patient's specific argument and repeats his former denial to the patient's self-characterization. He continues, "As for:: as: your present situation, it is not that you do not have a source of satisfaction, it's just that it is not ideal (. .), not what your heart-mind wants it to be." To this, the doctor finally gets a wholehearted acknowledgement from the patient (turn 93).

The doctor's concluding words in this long turn (turn 93) are almost an exact repetition of what he says at the beginning of the turn. But at the beginning of the turn, despite several tacit attempts from the doctor to get the patient's confirmation, the patient fails to respond. It is true that in certain conversational contexts, lack of response may imply confirmation. However, since the doctor's comment here contradicts the patient's previous self-evaluation (turn 91), the absence of confirmation suggests disagreement. Then we may ask why later the patient gives a completely different response to similar statements. In fact, we may notice that a similar interactive pattern starts to appear. For instance, when the doctor finishes his sentence, "it's just that it is not ideal," he pauses a little, inviting the patient to respond. He fails, which is what happened at the beginning of the turn. Therefore, we may infer that the patient's positive response is not to this particular utterance, but to the utterance that follows, "not what your heart-mind wants it to be."

Therefore, when the patient says "yes, exactly," she means yes, her life and work are not going according to her heart's desire. The doctor's last sentence is shaped to make his point and at the same time to elicit an agreement from the patient. With this agreement, both the doctor's long turn of *kaidao* and the patient's experience are somewhat acknowledged. The feeling of things going against her heart's wishes echoes throughout the interaction. The typical characterization of this feeling has something to do with *xin* (heart-mind) and manifests in somatic, emotional, and social terms. Her very first complaint is heart vexed (*xinfan*). The patient reports "unhappy things happening in her everyday life"; she says that after some time her personal life still cannot be satisfactorily resolved, her heart-emotion "persistently [does] not flow smoothly" (*laoshi bu shuchang*). Later, she again claims her heart-emotion does not flow smoothly and freely and says that both her life and work "do not flow smoothly with her heart" (*bu tai shunxin*). Again, when the patient talks about her frustration at work, she says that she feels "very uncomfortable in the heart" (*xinli te bu shufu*) and "very frustrated" (*te wonang*). The patient, though coming to seek a *zhongyi* medical treatment, understands that her illness originates socially, resulting from the conflicts between her mindful heart's desire and social reality. She honestly believes that if her problems in life and work can be resolved satisfactorily, her illness would be cured.

However, the idea of "being not ideal" (*bu lixiang* 不理想) is more from the doctor's point of view. In a sense, the doctor believes that the patient focuses on something that is "ideal" rather than "real." This perspective of the doctor becomes obvious from the conversation that follows. The doctor also sees that the patient's illness has a clear social origin, and he also assumes that if the patient's social circumstance changes, her emotional and bodily experience will probably change, too. This is not just common sense but has been meticulously theorized in the *zhongyi* understanding of *shenti* (body-person), emotion, and illness. However, as a therapist in modern Chinese society, the doctor does not have the means to directly intervene into the patient's social relations, given that a person's social world involves practically far more complicated factors than a doctor is able to deal with. What he is able to do is to help the patient to "transform emotions and change perspectives" (*yiqing yizhi*). Sivin points out that the *zhongyi* doctor still has to make decisions: "When confronted with a withdrawn young woman, to encourage her to change her situation, or to deceive her so that she will accept it docilely."[36] In modern *zhongyi* practice, it is not as much to "deceive" a patient as to persuade her to step back from her narrow personal concerns to embrace a broader view of life. This tendency marked the doctor's discourse of *kaidao* (persuasions), in which we see the doctor frequently uses such abstract phrases as "human life" and "society." This difference in the negotiation between two different perspectives continues to the end of the conversation.

In turn 95 (see transcript segment 7.7 for 95–100), the patient once again insists that her unsolved social problem is the key to her illness. She argues eloquently with the doctor who throughout the interaction tries to persuade the patient to change her perspective. The patient insists that her problems remain unsolved, and even though she tries not to focus on them, they are her reality: "Since they are unsolved, you cannot stop thinking about them, right?" Clearly, the patient shares the *zhongyi* assumption that "excessive thinking" (*silu guodu* 思虑过度) results in medical problems. She insists that she cannot help from dwelling on these problems; they are part of her social reality. The doctor chooses not to directly address the patient's rhetorical question and replies, "It is impossible to have everything go completely according to one's wishes" (96). By not addressing the patient's question, the doctor avoids discussing her argument that her social problems need to be solved before she is able to change her focus in life. He then turns to challenge her basic complaint that things fail to go according to how she wants them to go. As mentioned above, the patient has expressed her frustration as "not going smoothly according to her heart-emotion's desire" (*bu shunxin*) or "not conforming to her liking" (*bu he xinsi* 不合心思). The doctor's challenge is legitimate and to the point. He does not directly comment on the patient's behavior as it is but resorts again to a generalized statement about human life. He, on the one hand, tacitly criticizes the patient as self-centered, suggesting that the reason that the patient's problems remain unsolved is because she expects the impossible, but on the other hand, he avoids the patient's possible rejection.

The subsequent response from the patient shows that the patient does hear the doctor's comments as criticism, and she tries to defend herself in response. Since the criticism is only implied by a generalized statement, a straight forward rejection does not seem appropriate, particularly when the statement rings so true in Chinese common sense, which emphasizes relatedness and interdependence of the members within a society. The patient defends herself by saying that she only wishes that her problems could be solved perfectly (*yuanman de* 圆满地). The hesitations and pauses at the beginning of her sentence indicate that the patient feels difficulty in challenging the doctor's criticism. Before she finishes her sentence, the doctor quickly grasps the word the patient used "perfectly" (*yuanman de*) and cuts in: "You can on::ly talk about re:latively satisfactory. Completely satisfied (.)? That's not possible." By this, the doctor finally gets the patient to admit: "I have probably expected too:: much " (99).

After the patient finishes her turn, the doctor waits for about one second before he responds, showing little eagerness to comment on the patient's newly acquired insight. We may think that the doctor's perspective is finally accepted by the patient and that he probably would show his agreement with the patient in his response. Yet, when he starts to respond, he says "no" (*bushi*), which seemingly contradicts the patient's statement. Then, what can we make out of this particular denial, "*bushi*"? We have to look at the interactional sequence that directly leads to the patient's utterance in 99. Turn 96 can be read as a criticism of the patient, accusing her of being unrealistic. Facing this criticism, the patient's choice is either to accept or deny it. We see that in turn 97 the patient makes an effort to deny the criticism by qualifying her position. However, the patient's choice of "perfectly" (*yuanman de*) happens to serve the doctor's point, and the doctor quickly takes the opportunity to launch a further criticism that the patient is being unrealistic. Now, we see that the patient's utterance of 99 is a reluctant acceptance of a criticism. The doctor might at this point also notice that he has been a little too harsh in the past two turns. Then "*bushi*" could be read as "no, I am not saying this" or "no, this is not what I mean." Then, following this denial, the doctor is obliged to deal with what he really means to offset the image of being unsympathetic. We see that after the doctor's "*bushi*," there are many hesitations, repetitions, pauses, and false starts, indicating that the doctor is not comfortable with his seemingly irreconcilable positions. He is trying to formulate a coherent utterance that is both consistent with the idea that he has been making throughout the conversation that the patient is being unrealistic and unpractical and with the denial that he is not being unsympathetic or not understanding.

The doctor's "no" can also be read in a slightly different way. From the perspective of conversational structure, when a person makes a negative evaluation of herself, it projects a constraint on the next turn and makes it relevant to the evaluation. Normally, after a negative self-evaluation, a denial is preferred. The patient's turn 99 is clearly a negative self-evaluation, though it is in agreement with the doctor's evaluation. The doctor is obliged to contradict at least in form. We have seen throughout the conversation, that this doctor is sensitive to the patient's negative self-evaluations and tends to contradict them whenever they appear. This happens similarly in the exchange of turns 91 and 92, though the contradiction was really meant by the doctor in that exchange.

Again, in his turn 100, the doctor resorts to the generalized point of view and uses "I think" to make his argument a part of his personal observation and experience. He emphasizes, "Wherever you go, there will be unhappy things. . . . As long as there are people, there are human relations to deal with." He then comes to a conclusion, which is the central theme of his *kaidao* (persuasion) and the idea he has been hammering at throughout the course of the conversation with the patient. The doctor points out that humans are social beings living in connection with others, and therefore conflicts of personal desires and interest are inevitable; "the question is how to deal with them. The key lies with the individual herself." The doctor encourages the patient to step out of her small world, to accept imperfectness as the way of the world, and to find a way to adjust to her environment and make the most out of it. The doctor's emphasis on the statement "The key lies with the individual herself" carries the double power of both criticism and encouragement by putting both the responsibility of being ill and the responsibility of getting well on the patient.

In addition to his role as a medical doctor, the doctor positions himself as a member of society who takes the point of view opposite to the patient's throughout the entire interaction. The opposite positions of the doctor and patient are evident in their self-presentations. The patient's voice is marked with personal pronouns "I" and "my," while the doctor's constant references to "human being" and "human society" lends him the voice of society. He tries to persuade the patient to examine the appropriateness and practicality of her own claims on society. Such examination requires the patient to step out of her "self" and assume the perspective of a culturally defined "wise and mature" person, who is able to assess a "situation" from *within* and *without* and "attune" her body-person accordingly to the flow of her social and natural world.

Transcript Segment 7.7

---

95. P: *y ushí xiànshí de shìr::*
    lǎo jiějué bù lǐ:ǎo ba: (.5) zìj
    xiǎng xiǎngkāi le yě xiǎng bu
    kāi: (. .) mm: jiějué bù lǐ:ǎo ah:
    z :ng xiǎ:ng zhèige wèntí ah::

96. D: *bù k néng wánquán dōu*
    héhu zìj ah: (.5) de xiǎngfǎ ah

97. P: *k : e: w : xi::ǎng (. .) yàoshi*
    néng yuánmǎn ji jué zhè liǎng
    f'iǎngmiàn de wèntí:=

98. D: *= zh néng shuō b jiǎo:*
    b jiǎo mǎnyì: n yào wán:quán
    mǎnyì (.) shì bù k néng de

99. P: *w k néng yāoqiú tài:gāo le*
    ba:: (1.0)

100. D: *búshi:: qísh: qíshí (.5)*
     shèhuì (. .) shèhuì shíjì:
     shēnghuó shíjì: w xiǎng (.8)
     dōu zhèyàng (.5) dào nǎr dōu
     y u bù:: yúkuài de shìqing (. .)
     ***dōuyǒu** rénjì guānxì wèntí*
     *(.) n **suànsuan** ba:: **méiyǒu***
     méiy u rénjì guānxì de wèntí
     zh yao y u rén shēnghuó de
     *dìfang(.) **dōu** y u rénjì guānxì*
     *(.) jiùshi: z nme **chùli** hǎo(. .)*
     *guānjiàn zài **zìjǐ:** ((Long*
     silence while the doctor
     is finishing writing the
     prescription.))

101. D: *bǎozhèng n néng hǎo āh:*

102. P: *nà jiù tài hǎo le ha::*
     h::((laugh))

103. D: *w men qiáobìng jiù y u*
     zhèi ge bǎwò (1.) yào bu=

104. P: *=tīng nín zhème shuō::w de*
     bìng jiù hǎo yí bànr le ha::h::
     ((laugh))

---

95. P: Sometimes, the problems of real life
    remain unsolved: uh: (.5), even though
    you yourself want to stop dwelling on
    them, you just can't help (. .) um: Since
    they are not solved uh: you just can not
    stop thinking about the problems, right?

96. D: It is simply impossible to have
    everything go completely according to
    your wish uh: (.5)

97. P: Bu: u: t I: thi::nk (. .) if only I'll
    be able to perfectly solve these two
    problems of my life:=

98. D: =You can on::ly talk about relatively:
    relatively satisfactory: Completely
    satisfactory? (.) That's not possible.

99. P: Well:: I have probably expected too:
    much (1.0)

100. D: No:: actual: actually (.5) society
     (. .) social reality: life reality: I think
     (.8) is all like this (.5) **Wherever you
     go**, there will be un::happy things (. .)
     there are problems of interpersonal
     relations (.) You *just thi::nk* about it::
     no place where you do not have to deal
     with interpersonal relationship (. .) As
     long as there are people (.) there are
     interpersonal relations (4.) The question
     is how to **handle** them (.) The key lies
     with the individual **oneself**. ((Long
     silence while the doctor is finishing
     writing the prescription.))

101. D: I guarantee you will get better, oka::y?

102. P: That will be really good. ha::h::
     ((laugh))

103. D: When we look at the illness, we have
     this assurance (1.) Otherwise=

104. P: = Just listening to what you just said::
     my illness is already half cured. Ha::h::
     ((laugh))

The source of persuasion that a *zhongyi* doctor relies on is eminently cultural. With Western psychotherapy, choices of conflict and confrontation may be viewed as the preferred mechanism in solving problems. "The patient is encouraged to express the feeling, to gratify the desire, and to remove the suppression."[37] However, with *zhongyi*, the patient is encouraged to contain (*baorong* 包容), dissolve (*huajie* 化解), and then transform (*zhuanhua* 转化) the conflicts by emphasizing the connectedness of self and others, individual and society, human being and the myriad things of the world. What is emphasized is the sense of unity and harmony with nature and the world. From this enlightened point of view, the ups and downs of life are viewed as "the waxing and waning of the moon," or in Joseph Needham's words, the "orderly processes of changes."[38] The doctor calls this "the sense of ordinariness" (*pingchang xin* 平常心), which is viewed as important for a healthy and mature person and is frequently emphasized in *zhongyi* counseling. *Zhongyi* practice is not just a way to heal, but also a process to transmit cultural values and social ideology.

Arthur and Joan Kleinman argue that efficacy is "an altered body-self, but also an altered flow of relationships, an altered world."[39] In this sense, the path to ultimate efficacy involves redefining reality, reorientating focus, and reordering the experience of local worlds. The patient in this case presents herself as a passive victim of her social environment from the beginning. From her perspective, her heart-emotion vexation and physical and emotional symptoms all result from her stagnant personal life and her stressful and unsympathetic working environment, and in turn, her emotional and bodily dysfunctions impede her social performance. She referred to this situation as a "vicious cycle." Her seeking *zhongyi* help is an effort to break the cycle by dealing with her emotional and bodily experience. However, she maintains that the unresolved social problems are the sources of her suffering, about which she cannot do anything. Although having recognized the social factors in the patient's suffering, the doctor insists that the patient herself must make a difference. From the doctor's perspective, his patient needs to rethink her own "heart-mind's" claim on society. Seeing that transformation of the patient's experience relies very much on her ability to reassess her situation and readjust her social relations, the doctor makes every effort to persuade the patient to change her attitude and see things from a different perspective. As shown at the end of the conversation, the doctor and the patient achieve some sort of alignment when the patient admits that she might have expected too much (see turn 99 in transcript segment 7.7) and claims jocosely that her illness is half cured just by listening to the doctor (turn 104). The patient and doctor part with a shared expectation that the prescribed herbs and an "attuned" attitude would help improve the patient's health. Both the doctor and patient understand that the process of "attuning" has just started, and the ultimate efficacy of restoring health demands diligent and continuous efforts from both the patient and the doctor.

As analyzed above, for a *qingzhi* (emotion-related) disorder, defined as "illness due to disordered emotions" (*yi qing bing zhe* 以情病者), *zhongyi* doctors particularly emphasize the importance of the patients' ability to "transform their emotions and change their perspectives" (*yiqing yizhi*). They assume that changes in one's attitude and behavior have physiological outcomes and vice versa. Therefore, "talking" as persuasion or manipulation of emotions is also an integrated part of *zhongyi* therapy, which is very often accepted as merely herbal therapy. However, *zhongyi* "talking" is not meant to be a "talk therapy" of the Western psychological counseling, and it should not be judged as such. It has to be understood in the light of the whole clinical process of *tiao*, aiming at adjusting multiple dimensions of the patient's experience, including prescribing medicinal herbs, and persuading the patient to "transform emotions and change perspectives." This analysis of the interaction between the doctor and patient could be elaborated into a sociocultural critique, in which the doctor can be seen as embodying the hegemony of established social orders and thus instrumental to social control. Such an analysis demands a further distance from the nitty-gritty nature of everyday clinical work perceived primarily as clinical actions against illnesses by both doctor and patient and an interpretation at a higher level of structural abstractions. Such a project could be a next step. Additionally, the transcribed data of naturally occurring clinical interaction is readily accessible to other interested scholars who may attempt to carry out a different type of analysis.

Finally, this chapter has empirically documented how the doctor and patient engage each other in determining the meaning of a particular illness and negotiating the path to efficacy. It is implied that a microanalytically oriented ethnography can provide unique empirical insights to complement the understandings derived from the more conventional approach of participant observation. In recent anthropological accounts of Chinese medicine, the detailed descriptions of observed cases and anecdotes and recorded experience reported to the researchers by informants help provide sophisticated pictures of *zhongyi* practice in time and place. However, given that a clinical encounter is fundamentally a face-to-face interaction, without considering its interactional aspect, our understanding of this "practice-oriented" healing system is incomplete. Even with the detailed description and analysis of the clinical process of *kanbing* (looking at illness) offered by Farquhar,[40] we still would "not know exactly how Chinese medical doctors get from patients' complaints to the prescription of specific drugs."[41] Here, microanalysis that relies on the actions and interactions of the participants themselves for analytical resources may offer the promise to trace how a particular syndrome type is defined and a therapeutic action is determined in a real episode of clinical encounter.

VIII

Conclusion

This book has offered an ethnographic account of how emotion-related disorders (*qingzhi bing* 情志病) are construed, constructed, treated, and experienced in the context of Chinese medicine, or *zhongyi* in contemporary China. I have structured my description in a way more or less matching the Chinese habit of defining a situation, that is, beginning with a broader context and gradually narrowing down to more specific observations. I start with a historical perspective of transformations of Chinese medicine, then move to the situated discussions of Chinese perceptions of body-person (*shenti* 身体), emotion (*qing* 情), emotion-related disorders (*qingzhi bing*), and finally to an analysis of a specific *zhongyi* clinical moment of attuning (*tiao* 调).

First of all, to make sense of the Chinese experience of being ill and being healed, we must "consider the presence of bodies."[1] Yet "the bodies" that the Chinese medicine works on and the Chinese patients experience are constructed differently from the Western commonsensical and bioscientific notion of body. They do not entail the distinction between mind and body or soma and psyche. The meaning and experience of a *qingzhi* disorder and its *zhongyi* treatment, then, must be interpreted within the Chinese conceptual and experiential world of lived body-person (*shenti*) which is, at the same time, emotive, moral, and visceral, and in relation to the embodied cultural values of everyday life. The concept of somatization by virtue of its dualistic presupposition has serious limitations in understanding Chinese embodied experience.

In presenting *qingzhi* disorders as Chinese experience, I explored in chapter 3 the Chinese conception and experience of *shenti* (body-person): how the Chinese world of *shenti* is patterned and shaped by cultural values and sensibilities that are deeply rooted in the bodily practice of everyday life. I particularly discussed the salient Chinese aesthetic values and sensibilities of flowing and connecting (*tong* 通), degree and position (*du* 度), and harmony (*he* 和) in shaping and giving meanings to the Chinese experience of being ill and being healed. I showed that the ordinary Chinese in their daily practices are oriented to a deeply embodied aesthetic order, which helps define *qingzhi* disorders as those characterized by stagnation, excessiveness, and disharmony in all the aspects of the local world. To make sense of Chinese *qingzhi* disorders, then, we have to attend to the "felt quality" of this world.

Second, the knowledge and practice of *zhongyi* is rooted in an epistemological tradition different from that of the paradigm of biomedicine that privileges a language of anatomic structures and reductive causality that characterizes a disease as a discrete entity. *Zhongyi*, however, privileges a language of process and transformation that describes a "syndrome pattern" (*zheng* 证) as a contingent state of dynamic relations in a pathological process. From functions of the visceral systems, to manifested bodily symptoms, to emotional-mental experience, and to natural and social environment, *zhongyi* physiology reveals a ceaseless continuum of process and transformation. The effect of a therapeutic intervention at any particular point of this continuum can be eventually transferred to other aspects of the body-person according to this physiology. Then, *zhongyi* healing entails a process of carefully studying and discerning the changes and relations of illness manifestations in time and space and using whatever technology is available—medicinal, psychological, and social—to manipulate the clinical dynamics and relations in order to enable a desirable development. This therapeutic process is best summarized as *tiao* (attuning).

Third, *zhongyi* healing should also be understood and analyzed as interactional phenomena in actual clinical work. *Zhongyi* is understood by doctors as "the science of practice" (*shijian de kexue* 实践的科学). *Zhongyi* theories and the accumulated knowledge of healing (*shijian jingyan* 实践经验) cannot be separated from actual clinical judgments and choices and ultimately the effects of the clinical work. As Farquhar points out, *zhongyi* knowledge is "quintessentially embodied and transmitted in the moment of clinical practice."[2] It follows from this that a close examination of what actually goes on and what is actually accomplished within the clinical process could be particularly informative to our understanding of *zhongyi* clinical practice. In addition, the participation of the patient is intrinsic to effective therapeutic practice. This is particularly significant in the *zhongyi* context. Yet, as I mentioned in chapter 7, Chinese medicine has not been studied empirically as actual social practice in its interactional context. Without considering the interactional aspect, our understanding of this practice-oriented healing system is incomplete.

As my analysis in chapter 7 demonstrates, a microanalitically oriented ethnography offers a vantage point from which to look at the *zhongyi* clinical practice of looking at an illness (*kanbing*). It provides empirical insights into many important theoretical issues of *zhongyi* practice. *Zhongyi* doctors and patients both emphasize the importance of accumulated experience through practice (*jingyan*) for a doctor in clinical practice, whereas in biomedicine the latest scientific knowledge and techniques are more revered. The long years of a doctor's experience are frequently in the*i* clinics. A legitimate question is how *jingyan* comes into play in an actual process of "differentiating syndromes and determining therapies." A close look at actual clinical interaction shows that the doctor's *jingyan* is deployed in his perception of the clinical situations in interactional forms, in his ability to make connections and assessment of symptoms, and very importantly, in his ways of engaging the patient. *Jingyan* is not only the accumulated knowledge that relates the doctor to a particular syndrome pattern and an herbal formula, but also the accumulated life experience that relates the doctor to the person who is suffering.

Since *Zhongyi* clinical process is characterized as "looking at illness" by both doctor and patient, an examination of the actual interaction that takes place in clinical practice offers a way to study how doctor and patient engage each other and bring their own insights to bear on the illness. As my analysis in chapter 7 shows, it is through the interactions between the doctor and patient that a particular *zhongyi* syndrome type emerges or is defined and a particular therapeutic method is determined. The microanalysis in chapter 7 empirically documents how the doctor and patient orient themselves to each other and negotiate the meanings of the illness and the path to efficacy.

Zhongyi practice is also recognized as having a holistic perspective (*zhengti guan* 整体观) that sees an illness as a disorder of body-person in relation to the social and natural environment. Very often the *zhongyi* holistic perspective is discussed in an abstract way as part of a theoretical discourse on the unity of human and nature. We rarely see how this holistic perspective is reflected in the clinical process. With a closer look at the actual clinical interaction, we can see that the connection of the patient's social environment, emotional experience, and physical suffering is assumed by both doctor and patient and is actively evoked in clinical actions and interactions. We can also see that the holistic principle is actually a practical guide in the *zhongyi* clinical work of differentiating syndromes and determining therapies.

This raises some very important questions. Does *zhongyi* address emotional complaints? How does *zhongyi* handle the emotional aspects of the patient's suffering? The impression that we get from many discussions of *zhongyi* and Chinese medical culture in general is that Chinese tend to emphasize physical discomfort rather than emotional complaints.[3] *Zhongyi* is said to conceptualize emotional disorders as physical illnesses and to treat them as such. Yet, as I showed in my microanalysis of a clinical interaction, it is obvious that, for treating *qingzhi* disorders, *zhongyi* does address the patient's emotional and social difficulties as well as her bodily dysfunctions. In fact, the microanalytically oriented study can be used as a tool of discovery. I myself was surprised, when I was transcribing the actual clinical interactions, at how much emphasis the patient put on her emotional disturbance and social difficulties and how much effort the doctor actually made to address the patient's social and emotional problems. Still, the question remains, why the fact that emotional aspects in *zhongyi* clinical work, which seems so obvious, has escaped analytical and ethnographic attention.

One possible reason is that the forms, concerns, and techniques of *zhongyi* counseling, as it is shown in chapter 7, are radically different from those of the standard Western psychological counseling. Comparing the framework of the Western "talk therapy" to *zhongyi* clinical contexts, the *zhongyi* doctor's approach resembles more of an informal persuasion by a close friend or family member than a professional exploration of the patient's inner emotional conflicts. This approach may seem less professional and effective, and therefore is not recognized as "really" dealing with the patient's emotional problems. However, as my analysis shows, the *zhongyi* "talking" or "counseling" is not meant to be a "talk therapy." It has to be understood in the light of the whole clinical process of "attuning" (*tiao*), which aims at adjusting multiple dimensions of the patient's experience, including persuading the patient to "transform emotions and change perspectives." Neither the doctor nor the patient assumes that a *qingzhi bing* is an illness exclusively in emotion or in mind, and "talking" will be the only legitimate way to heal. On the contrary, both the doctor and the patient assume that a *qingzhi bing* has social, emotional, and physical dimensions and various aspects of the intervention, such as an herbal prescription, an attuned attitude, change of behavior or the social environment, all have a stake in the transformation of experience in the body-person. Such a process of attuning has distinctive cultural meanings, and *zhongyi* talking should not be analyzed and judged separately from the cultural context of the whole clinical process of attuning. I do believe that a comparative investigation between the attuning and Western psychotherapy may generate some very interesting insights in understanding how emotion-related disorders are constructed and managed in Chinese society and in the Western cultures, but that has to be left for a future study.

When asked why *zhongyi* still enjoys such popularity in today's China when biomedical technology, compared with *zhongyi* practice, is equally available and affordable to the general population, one of the most frequently given answers is that *zhongyi* fits China's "national conditions" (*guoqing*) and is therefore liked by the majority of people. My interpretation of this is that *zhongyi* as an indigenous health care system shares with its patients a system of cultural values and orientations that recognize the incessant circulation between the physiological, the psychological, and the social. As discussed previously, *zhongyi* constructions such as *qingzhi* disorders offer a culturally meaningful form of suffering for Chinese patients and practical methods to cope with a lived body that falls out of order. My study has clearly illustrated this aspect of *zhongyi*.

However, there is still more that I would like to elaborate about Chinese experience of emotion-related disorders and Chinese medicine. Some are important issues that I have touched upon here and there, but have not systematically explored, for example the issue of *zhongyi* efficacy. We may say that *zhongyi* efficacy partially derives from *zhongyi's* cultural legitimacy. Yet, the question of medical efficacy: how it is evaluated and how it plays out in *zhongyi* practice and the *zhongyi* industry in today's China is far more complicated and certainly deserves "multidimensional approaches" to address it.[4]

Effectiveness of treatment (*liaoxiao* 疗效) is claimed by *zhongyi* professionals as the primary factor that *zhongyi* relies on for its success in the modern era. However, there has been little effort to address the question of how efficacy is constructed in *zhongyi* clinical contexts. What are *zhongyi's* criteria for determining efficacy? Have these criteria changed over time? How do the dynamics of integrating *zhongyi* with biomedicine influence the way *zhongyi* evaluates efficacy? Particularly, in recent years, the country's commitment to modernizations and overall engagement in the market economy have transformed Chinese social life in a significant way. Have these sociohistorical developments changed the basic terms on which *zhongyi* evaluates its efficacy or on which *zhongyi* is itself evaluated for efficacy? These are some of the questions that deserve further research.

To modernize *zhongyi* or to make *it* scientific (*zhongyi kexuehua*) has been a quest for generations of *zhongyi* professionals since the 1920s, yet these professionals also realize that simply applying the bioscientific standards and procedures to *the* practice and its efficacy is extremely difficult if not completely fruitless (Zhen et al. 1990:435–438). For example, to determine scientific efficacy of a simple herbal formula in the context of *zhongyi* would be a formidable task. There are too many variables that need to be controlled, considering how it is used in the actual clinical situation. A plant in itself does not mean much, and its particular effect needs to be understood as a result of interactions with other plants within the formula. A doctor almost always adds some additional ingredients to, and subtracts some from, the existing formula according to a particular case. Furthermore, the amount of each herbal element, the geographic origin of the plants, and the methods of processing and decocting the plants are all subject to manipulation. Therefore, even though each element can be tested separately for its pharmacological quality, the efficacy of a particular *zhongyi* formula is far from determined. In addition to all of this complexity, *zhongyi* holds that a particular patient's psycho-physiological disposition and his or her health condition at the particular time also influence the effectiveness of a therapy. In fact, efficacy is a much broader concept than just scientifically assessed effectiveness of a medicine.

Zhongyi, because it lies outside the paradigm of the modern biosciences, has been constantly questioned for its scientific value. At the same time, because of this, it is difficult for any scientific method to simply falsify or confirm the claims that *zhongyi* makes, unless we completely alter the basic terms and clinical conditions under which *it* works. Interestingly, *zhongyi* is able to actively exploit its conceptual incompatibility with science and negotiate its very prosperous presence in the modern age of science and technology. In this, *zhongyi* demonstrates its "historical toughness."[5] On the one hand, *it* engages science in producing and advertising a scientifically legitimate modern practice and industry, observable in *zhongyi* education, hospitals equipped with newly developed bioscience technology, and a booming industry of *zhongyi* patent medicine. On the other hand, *zhongyi* continues to evoke a different cultural modality quintessentially embodied in the "traditional" technology of differentiating syndrome patterns and determining therapies (*bianzheng lunzhi*) coupled with decocting herbs. When the paradigm shifts to *zhongyi* clinical practice, what is emphasized is practice and context, within which "science" is not absolute but rather debatable, contestable, and appropriable.

Transcription Conventions Used in the Text

I. The pinyin system is used in Chinese transcription. In CA done on English, punctuation marks are conventionally used to indicate intonation. Since Chinese is a tonal language, it is not necessary to use a separate system to indicate intonation. Punctuation is not used at all in the Chinese transcription. However, to make the translation easier to understand, punctuation marks are used for grammar in the English translation of the transcript.

II. The symbols used in the transcription are of standard notations developed in conversation analysis and used in most conversation analytical literature.

//	indicates the onset of overlapping utterances.
::	indicates that the sound followed by colons is lengthened.
=	is used at the end of one line and the beginning of another, indicates that no time elapsed between two lines of utterances.
(.)	(each dot in parentheses) indicates a pause of about one-tenth of a second.
(0.0)	indicates duration of pauses or silence in seconds.
(word)	indicates that the transcriber is not sure that the expression that appears in the parentheses is exactly what is said.
((word))	indicates transcriber's remarks.
word	indicates sound louder than normal speech.
word	indicates sound much louder than normal speech.
°word°	indicates sound uttered at low volume.

Notes

CHAPTER 1

1. The same category of illness is sometimes referred to as *shenzhi bing* 神志病 or *shen bing* 神病 (mind-related disorders). *Qingzhi* 情志, commonly translated as "emotions," specifically refers to the *zhongyi* concept of '*qiqing*' 七情 (seven emotive or mental activities): *xi* 喜 (joy), *nu* 怒 (anger), *you* 忧 (worry/anxiety), *si* 思 (thinking/longing), *bei* 悲 (sadness/grief), *kong* 恐 (fear), *jing* 惊 (fright). A detailed analysis of *qingzhi* is provided in chapter 4.

2. Zhang Jiebin in his book *Lei Jing* 类经 (Comments on Internal Classics 1624) listed twenty-nine comments under the heading of *qingzhi bing*. See also Sivin 1995 for the discussion of a group of disorders collected under the heading *qingzhi* (emotions) in Wu Kun's *Yifang Kao* 医方考 (*Research on Medical Formulas*) (1584).

3. Jackson 1994:211.

4. Yap 1974.

5. See Tseng et al. 1995; Cheng 1995; Yang 1995.

6. Kleinman 1986.

7. See Lucas and Barret 1995 for a discussion of psychiatric primitivism.

8. Scheid 2002:13.

9. See Csordas 1994.

10. See Desjailais 1992, for the critique of symbolic approach to culture in anthropology.

11. Brownell 1995:15.

12. Jenkins and Valient 1994.

13. Ots 1990:12.

14. Desjarlais 1992:71

15. See Good and Good 1982.

16. Frake 1961.

17. Browner et al. 1988.

18. Also talked about as referential meaning. See also White 1993.

19. Good and Good 1982:143.

20. Good 1977:27.

21. See Lock and Scheper-Hughes 1990.

22. See Taussig 1980; Young 1982.

23. Scheper-Hughes1992.

24. Kleinman and Kleinman 1991, 1995.

25. See Frankel 1983, Mishler 1984; West 1984; Heath 1984.

26. There are many different approaches to discourse analysis. My microanalytical approach draws mostly from conversation (talk-in-interaction) analysis (see Atkinson and Heritage 1984) and interactional sociolinguistics (see Goffman 1964, 1974, 1981; Gumperz 1982). More discussion is given in chapter 6.

27. See David L. Hall and Roger Ames (1987) for detailed discussion of Chinese cosmological assumptions that are uncommon to the Western philosophic reflections.

28. See Farquhar 1994.

29. Good 1994.

30. Wu (1982:285) discusses the use of psychotherapy in classical Chinese medicine and points out that the concepts of 'health' and 'health care' in classic texts emphasized the interrelations between a person's state of mind and that of his/her health. For the past two decades, numerous publications on zhongyi psychology (zhongyi xinlixue 中医心理学) or heart-body medicine (xinshen yixue 心身医学) have appeared, for example, Wang 1986, Dong et al. 1987, Zhang 1995, Dong 2001, Dong and Li 2003.

31. See Cheung et al. 1981; Kleinman 1980, 1986; Kleinman and Mechanic 1981; T. Y., Lin 1983; Tseng 1975.

32. According to Zheng Yanping at al. (1986:237), the language many Chinese depressive patients use does not fit comfortably into the two patterns of psychologization and somatization suggested by some researchers in the West (e.g., Marsella 1980; Good and Kleinman 1985). Chinese patients may use language that evokes bodily images or experience, but it is certainly not somatic in opposition to psychological.

33. Other forms of traditional treatment likely to be mentioned by patients are acupuncture, massage, and qigong (meditative) exercise and therapy. One patient whom I interviewed told me that once her family took her to the countryside to be treated by a shaman doctor.

34. See Sivin 1995.

35. Scheper-Hughes and Lock 1987:9.

36. Ames 1993:105.

37. Commonly translated as "spirit" or "mental."

38. See also Hall and Ames 1987:20.

39. See Farquhar 1994:18.

40. See Lin and Eisenberg 1985. From many psychiatrists working in Chinese society, zhongyi is understood as having a somato-psychic approach to treatment of mental illness, that is, treating mentally ill through manipulation of physiological functions. Such an approach is often cited as an obstacle to the development of psychiatry in China.

41. See Cheung 1982, 1989; Kleinman 1977, 1982, 1986; Lin 1985; Tseng 1983; Zhang 1989.

42. See Kleinman 1977, 1980; Leff 1981; Tseng 1975.

43. Jenkins and Valient 1994:173. According to Kleinman (1986:149), somatization is "the substitution of somatic preoccupation for dysphoric affect in the form of complaints of physical symptoms and even illness." Later, he redefines the concept as "the normative expression of personal and social distress in an idiom of bodily complaints and medical help-seeking" (1986:2). Others define it as "expression style or idiom of emotion" (Zheng at al. 1989:240), "illness pictures in which bodily symptoms are overly dominant," and "embraces displaced psychosocial distress" (Fabrega 1990:1). The concept presupposes an ontological distinction between the somatic and the psychological and involves "a postulate about the correspondence and association between changes in the body as versus the mind and behavior" (Fabrega 1990: 654).

44. Jenkins and Valient 1994-173

45. Kleinman 1980:146.

46. F. M., Cheung 1995:166.

47. Cheng 1995.

48. Tseng 1974.

49. See Cheung 1995; Young 1989; Zheng et al. 1986.

50. In recent years, China has made mental health a public health priority and developed many social and mental health programs (Cohen, Kleinman, Saraceno 2002:15). Yet, these psychiatric-oriented programs and services rarely bring in Chinese medical expertise in their design. Even the community-based Shanghai model aimed at both treatment and rehabilitation does not consider Chinese medicine as relevant. Yet many psychiatric patients, as I observed during my fieldwork, do seek *zhongyi* help for treatment of their illnesses.

51. In fact, therapeutic manipulation of emotions and thoughts by *zhongyi* doctors was documented in early Chinese medical classics. See Sivin 1995; Wu 1982. More detailed information is provided in chapters 3 and 4.

52. See Hsu 1999; Scheid 2002; Sivin 1987; Unschuld 1985.

53. See also Scheid 2002.

54. Hsu 1999.

55. Scheid 2002:2.

56. Ibid., 263.

57. People's Medical Publishing House:139.

58. Although the typical patients of Shenjing Ke include those with neurological disorders and those with what Western medicine calls "psychological" or "psychiatric" problems, the distinction of different *ke* in a *zhongyi* hospital is not as significant as in a biomedical hospital. Such a distinction is significant to the doctors mostly in terms of different points of view or positions in approaching the same pathological reality. It is common that a patient consults different *ke* in one visit to the hospital, and the doctor and patient do not seem to have problems with different prescriptions since ideally these prescriptions aim at the same pathological conditions with a different emphasis.

59. I was particularly close to two student doctors, Dr. Huang and Dr. Lee. Huang had been a *zhongyi* doctor for five years in Hebei province before coming to Beijing for

further training. She offered to accompany me on my visits to patients. Lee was a graduate student from South Korea. She let me borrow her notes whenever I needed them. She was also a patient. I observed a couple of times when patients were not present, she asked the doctor to "look at her illness" and was prescribed herbal medicine for sleeping problems and low energy.

60. The opposite movement is less evident but definitely exists. Based on my observation, local doctors from provincial areas with special efficacy in treating certain difficult diseases are also invited to treat patients in larger hospitals in Beijing.

61. My friend, an instructor in a *zhongyi* college, insisted on paying the bills whenever we dined out, saying that she made more than I did. She explained that although her salary was nothing, by taking in patients privately she could make a couple of thousand Chinese yuan a month.

62. These sources include Farquhar 1994; Liu 1988; Ou et al. 199; 1992; Scheid 2002; Sivin 1987; and Chinese Terms in Traditional Chinese Medicine and Pharmacy (*Zhongyiyaoxue Mingci* 中医药学名词) 2004.

CHAPTER II

1. An experienced senior *zhongyi* doctor is frequently invited to attend group consultations, which usually include both *zhongyi* and *xiyi* doctors on difficult medical cases. Generally, the *zhongyi* doctors are the ones who are expected to move back and forth between two medical systems, while biomedical doctors are not expected to master *zhongyi* concepts and language.

2. According to my clinical observation in a *zhongyi* hospital, a doctor does not routinely order laboratory tests or examinations using penetrative imaging devices except on suspicion of serious organic diseases. For *zhongyi* intervention, the purpose of these tests and examinations is not strictly diagnostic in nature since the test result is not essential in determining the therapeutic principle or in choosing or designing the drug formula. Generally, the purpose is to determine whether or not there exists any serious organic problem that requires drastic intervention of biomedicine. Sometimes, patients ask for certain tests and examinations or biomedical drugs. Doctors usually go along with the requests in order to let the patients have peace of mind (*fangxin* 放心). However, in the hospital where I did my research there is a clear guideline regarding how much biomedicine a doctor can prescribe. Generally it should not exceed 15 percent of the total prescription. Occasionally, administrative personnel would come down to the clinics to check the records. Situations might be different in a clinic or hospital of integrated Chinese and Western medicine (*zhongxiyi jiehe* 中西医结合), where biomedical examinations and drugs are used more liberally. See Scheid 2002:95.

3. Since many hospitals of Chinese medicine also run a clinic of Western medicine, and biomedical hospitals normally have a Chinese medical section, patients sometimes choose to see both a biomedical doctor and a *zhongyi* doctor in the same visit to the hospital. There is also a form of practice officially called "integrative treatment of Chinese and Western medicine" (*zhongxiyi jiehe zhiliao* 中西医结合治疗), which is recognized as a practice seperate from either Chinese or Western medicine.

4. See Farquhar 1994.

5. According to the earliest oracle bone inscriptions in the Shang Dynasty (1766–1122 BCE), the character of *yi* 医 was etymologically composed of two parts, *yi* (illness, cure) and *wu* 巫 (divination). Later in the Zhou Dynasty (1122–772 BCE), the character was transformed into its contemporary form composed of cure and wine (*jiu* 酉) (see Tseng 1974). According to the earliest Chinese dictionary *Shuo Wen* 说文, *yi* means a person who cures illness with wines. In the Spring and Autumn of the Zhou Dynasty (770–476 BCE), *yi* (physician; medicine) and *wu* (shaman; divination) had became separate specializations listed in different official categories. Medical practice during this period "witnessed the beginning of an organization" (Hoisey and Hoisey 1993:55). According to *The Zhouli* 周礼 (*The Rite of Zhou*), at the top of the medical hierarchy were the *yishi* 医师 (master physicians), under whom there were also *shiyi* 食医 (physicians for nutrition), *jiyi* 疾医 (physicians for the cure of illness), *yangyi* 疡医 (physicians for treating wounds), and *shouyi* 兽医 (physicians for animals) (see Zhen et al. 1991).

6. Porkert (1974) refers to this healing system as the medicine of "systematic correspondence."

7. According to Sivin, "classic medicine does not refer to the theory and practice of a coherent group, but to the records left by the most literate and scholarly representatives of several traditions (1987:22–23).

8. It may sound like an oversimplification, but from the point of view of many senior doctors who lived through the years struggling for survival in the 1920s and 30s, the contrast between the current state of full legitimacy and official support and the past insecurity is real. The feeling is fully illustrated in the poem by Zhang Zanchen, a renowned senior doctor: "*Zhongyi* at the present is absolutely different from the past, like an ancient tree revived thriving green in Spring" (quoted in Li 1987:39).

9. Faquhar 1994:12.

10. According to Unschuld (1985), when Robert Morrison, the first Protestant missionary in China, and J. Livingston, a physician of the East India Company, opened a pharmacy and started to treat patients in Macao in 1820, Western medicine did not yet have much to offer. Their willingness to learn native healing techniques, in a certain sense, shows that "therapeutic knowledge available to Western physicians at the time was still not yet sufficient to occasion an attitude of superiority" (236). Unschuld also maintains that when Peter Parker, the first Protestant missionary with complete medical training, set up a clinic in Canton in 1835, "it was primarily minor surgical procedures, such as the removal of external tumors and the treatment of superficial ailments, as well as spectacular cataract operations, that quickly made him famous." See also Cai 1988:523.

11. See Hoizey and Hoizey 1993:150; Unschuld 1985:239. After the second Opium War, the Western powers' privileges in China were further confirmed and extended from the coastal treaty ports to the interior, where in forty years from 1860, 100 missionary hospitals were established (Zhen et al. 1991:411).

12. Quite a few influential reform-minded intellectuals and politicians of the time had once in their careers chosen to study Western medicine, including Sun Yat-sen and Lu Xun.

13. Quoted from Unschuld 1985:230.

14. The discourse of *xin* 新 (new) versus *jiu* 旧 (old) became a dominant rhetoric in the new culture movement (1914–19) with *xin* associated with things modern, progressive, and Western, and *jiu* with things outdated, backward, and traditional Chinese. The term *jiu yi* 旧医 (old medicine) referring to Chinese medicine was used profusely by those who argued for abolishing *zhongyi*. Yu Yunxiu in his *Revolution of Medicine* (1914) invariably referred to Chinese medicine as *jiuyi* that should be completely obliterated. He argued that "medicine was not to be divided into Chinese and Western, and the only meaningful division was 'new' from 'old/backward' (*yi wu fen zhong-xi, dan you xin-jiu eryi*. 医无分于中西, 但有新旧而已)." See Zhen et al. 1991:428–433.

15. Zhen et al. 1994:487.

16. Cai 1988:524.

17. Unschuld 1985:246–247.

18. *Different Schools of Chinese Medicine* (*Zhongyi Gejia Xueshuo* 中医各家学说) edited by Ren et al. (1994) identifies seven major schools (*xuepai* 学派) of medical thoughts in history. These are Hejian, Yishui, Danxi, Gongxie, Wenbu, Shanghan, and Wenbing.

19. Zhen et al. 1991:441.

20. Ibid., 490–492.

21. The Central National Institute was established in 1930 (Zheng et al. 1991).

22. See Zhen et al. 1991:499–528.

23. In fact, the argument to abandon or radically reform Chinese medicine was presented equally in patriotic terms if not more.

24. Quoted in Zhen et al. 1994:426.

25. See Scheid 2002:66–106.

26. The Chinese original is "Zhongguo yiyao xue shi yi ge weida de baoku, yingdang luli fajue, jiayi tigao 中国医药学是一个伟大的宝库, 应当努力发掘, 加以提高."

27. Until 1949, all kinds of infectious and parasitic diseases, such as plague, cholera, smallpox, tuberculosis, black water fever, malaria, and bilharzias had raged across the country. According to the statistics on twelve infectious diseases of 1947, about 1.3 million were infected and more than 100,000 people died. (Zhen, et al. 1991:540). In old China (before the founding of the PRC in 1949), there were only limited hospitals concentrated in main cities. Most Chinese did not have access to these rare medical resources. To improve health conditions for all the Chinese people became an urgent task for the new government. At the first National Conference on Public Health held in 1950, one year after the Communists took power, three objectives were set: health work should be aimed at the mass of workers, peasants, and soldiers; prevention should take priority; and Chinese and Western medicines should be united. See Hoizey and Hoizey 1993:176.

28. See Zhen et al. 1991:555–556; and Li 1987: 36–37. When the first hospital, the Red Hospital, was set up in 1927 in the Jingang Mountain Revolutionary Base, two of the three doctors were doctors of Chinese medicine. The division of practice was that *zhongyi* treated ordinary diseases with herbal medicine and the *xiyi* handled the external injuries. The Red Army also set up medical schools to teach basic biomedical knowledge and Chinese medicine. The use of both Western and Chinese medicine has been in practice since the Jingang Mountains period.

29. Bao Jingheng 1950 "Why Chinese medical doctors need further training," in *Jian Kang* Vol. 135, quoted in Zhen et al. (1991).

30. Unschult 1985:251.

31. See Zhen et al.1991:487–528. The *Guideline for Academic Standardization of National Medicine* (*Zhengli Guoyiyao Xueshu Biaozhun Dagang* 整理国医药学术标准大纲) was compiled and published by the Central Academy of National Medicine (Zhongyang Guoyi Guan 中央国医馆) in 1933. Later based on this guideline, the academy issued a document suggesting unifying *zhongyi* illness names with the Western illness names. In the 1930s, Western medicine was incorporated in the curriculum of many *zhongyi* shools. For example, courses such as anatomy, physiology, public hygiene, bacteriology, and pathology were taught in the North China Institute of National Medicine, established by renowned *zhongyi* physician, Shi Jinmo 施今墨, in 1932.

32. Scheid 2002:66.

33. Often simply referred to as *Neijing* (the Inner Classics).

34. *Hanshu: Yiwenzhi* 汉书:艺文志 (*Records of Han Dynasty: Bibliography of Art and Literature* 206 BCE–220 CA:) lists 868 volumes of medical treatises in 36 categories. Except for the *Huangdi Neijing*, all the others are lost. Several volumes of ancient medical works were excavated in the third Han tomb (dated 168 BCE) in Mawangdui in the 1970s. These works were not even listed in *Hanshu* and possibly antedated *Neijing*. *Neijing*, composed of two books, *Suwen* 素问 (*Basic Questions*) and *Lingshu* 灵枢 (*Divine Pivot*), covers various topics ranging from the relationship of a human being to his or her natural environment and discussion of human psychology, physiology, pathology, illness diagnosis, treatment, and prevention. Many important theoretical basics of today's *zhongyi* can be traced to this book. It is believed to be the product of a group of different authors at different times. Its compilation may have lasted for centuries, starting during the Warring State period (around 500 BCE). It did not take on its final form until Qin (221–207 BCE) and Han (206 BCE–23 CA). The book probably started as scattered texts, which were later added to, revised, and rearranged. The heterogenesis of the book is marked by repetitions and inconsistency in content and style. See Zhen et al. 1991; Hoizey and Hoizey 1993.

35. See Jiqun, Xu & Qingzhi, Wang 1985:1. Zhang Zhongjing (150–219 AD) is said "to creatively integrate the medical theories (li), methods (fa), formulas (fang), and drugs (yao)" in his book *Shanghai zabing Lun* (Discussion of Cold Damage and various disorders), and was therefore referred to as "*fangshu zhi zu*" 方书之祖 (the ancestor of formulas).

36. See Unschult 1985:250–251; 1992:54.

37. Scheid 2002:9.

38. Zhen 1991:100–110. See also Feng and Zhang 2004.

39. See Tian 2005 for information on *Yijing* and Chinese philosophic thought of *tongbian* (通变).

40. For example, *Neijing*'s statements about *mingmen* 命门 (gate of life) and *sanjiao* 三焦 (three burners) contradict completely the statements given in *Nanjing* 难经 (On Difficult Medical Issues), another canonical medical text published in Han period before Zhang Zhongjing's *Shanghan Lun*.

41. See also Scheid 2002:209–211.

42. Ames 1992.

43. Farqhuar 1994: 28.

44. Wang Qi (2003) examines the professional accomplishments of 112 renowned contemporary *zhongyi* doctors and their ways to become *da yi* 大医 (exemplary physicians). She noted that all of them emphasize the importance of memorizing *zhongyi* classic texts.

45. Sivin 1987:27.

46. While it is true that contemporary *zhongyi* education increasingly depends on the latest textbooks, the latest textbooks in Chinese medicine probably do not differ as much as in modern medicine from previous textbooks. The difference among various textbooks depends more on the purpose of the books, such that the textbooks written for students specializing in *zhongyi* are different from the textbooks that are written for students of biomedicine, in style, depth, detail, and language. Classic medical sources actually feature prominently in recent textbooks, where at the end of each chapter, relevant selected readings of classics (*wenxian xuandu* 文献选读 or *wenxian zhailu* 文献摘录) are provided in their original forms. Total translation of classic medical texts into modern Chinese has never been wholeheartedly carried out. The common practice is to publish the *yuanwen* 原文 (the original text) along with historical and linguistic notes and modern paraphrases. See also Farquhar 1994:28.

47. Farquhar 1994:29.

48. Sivin 1987:25.

49. Hall and Ames 1987:44.

50. In reading biographies of renowned *zhongyi* physicians, I notice that almost all of them have their favorite *zhongyi* classics that they claim help shape their own clinical work and that they tend to go back to frequently.

51. A discussion of this worldview can be found in chapter 3. For more information, see Hall and Ames 1987.

52. See Unshult, 1992-58. He suggests the possible existence of a fundamental dividing line between Chinese cognitive dynamics marked by "an expansion of knowledge, adding new to the old." And Western cognitive dynamics "characterized by a replacing of the old with the new."

53. See Farquhar's analysis of the relationship between past experience and present clinical actions in Chinese medicine. She argues, by evoking past experience, a doctor is drawing on the scholarly and clinical experience of his forbearers. He puts their insights into play when he decides they are appropriate to the specific case of the present; he modifies their formulae according to the present situation. "In doing so he both reanimates the experience of his forebears and makes his own contribution to a continuing process of accumulation" (1992:72–73).

54. Unshult (1985; 1992), Farquhar (1994), and Scheid (2002) all mentioned the influence of "dialectics" in shaping *zhongyi* knowledge in the 1950s and 1960s.

55. See *Zhongguo Keji Daobao* 中国科技导报 (Chinese Science and Technology) 1999;V7.

56. See "The speech given by senior *zhongyi* physicians Jiao Shude & Deng Tiatao" in *Xiandai Jiaoyubao* 现代教育报 (Modern Education) August 10, 2001. As was also reported recently on CCTV news (September 9, 2004), many *zhongyi* graduate students have a good knowledge of the English language and computer science but have little time for studying Chinese medicine. Some of them can hardly understand the introduction of *Bencao Gangmu* 本草纲目 (Outlines of Material Medica).

57. See a series of articles by Mao Jialing published in *Zhongguo Zhongyiyao Bao* 中国中医药报 (Chinese Medicine and Pharmacy Weekly) between January and May 2004.

58. *Zhongguo Zhongyiyao Bao* recently invited specialists from various fields to participate in "Zhongyi and Science Forum 2004."

59. See the recently published "Outline for the development of *zhongyi* clinical research" (*zhongyyi linchuang yanjiu fazhan gangyao* 中医临床研究发展纲要 1999–2015) drafted by the Division of Education of the State Zhongyiyao Administrative Bureau.

60. For example, the formula of *xiao chaihu tang* (decoction of blupeuri) is originally recorded in *Shanghan Lun* (Discussions of Cold Damage) and used for treating *shaoyang* (lesser yang) disorder. This specific formula has been used for thousands of years by Chinese physicians for its effectiveness in removing the heat, activating *qi* movement, and nourishing the stomach *yin*. In the 1970s, a Japanese pharmaceutical company started to manufacture the medicine based on this formula which was later clinically tested as having efficacy in treating chronic hepatitis. It was then used liberally to treat hepatitis in Japan. In the 1990s, reports came out that the manufactured Bupleuri could cause interstitial pneumonia that could result in death. See Feng et al. 2004: 32–34.

61. See the newspaper article by Wang, "Suping in *Jiankang Bao*" 健康报 (Health Weekly) December 10, 2003.

62. Translations are my own unless otherwise noted.

63. Farquhar 1994:20. See also Fauquhar 2002:41–77 on medicinal meals in contemporary China.

64. According to Wei, Yu, and Minghui Ren (1997:152), the major profit for hospitals comes from selling drugs. Hospitals are allowed to add 15 percent to the cost of purchased drugs. Hospitals tend to make more profit on self-produced drugs.

CHAPTER III

1. See Csordas 1990, 1994.

2. Roger Ames suggests that Chinese tradition is "eventful" rather than "essential," so gerunds are better than nouns for translating Chinese concepts. Hence *shenti* might be better rendered "bodying" (Personal communication 1997).

3. Desjarlais 1993.

4. Lutz 1988:54.

5. Lee 1996:437. See also Kleinman 1980, 1986; F. Cheung 1981; Ots 1990. Kleinman sees somatization as a basic feature of illness construction in Chinese culture. Susan Brownell 1994, following Kleinman's concept of somatization, claims "somatization has characterized Chinese culture since ancient times" (238).

6. See Kleinman 1980, 1986; Ots 1990, 1994.

7. Ots 1990:23.

8. See Zhang 1989. Many Western and Western-trained psychiatrists believe that Chinese medicine has never seen emotion or emotional disorders as "the legitimate domain of medicine," and thus doctors of Chinese medicine do not take treating emotional disorders as their responsibility.

9. It is very common that a patient presents a banner to the clinic or doctor who has successfully treated him or her. I saw banners presented to the doctors who were specialists on mental disorders, but in the fertility clinics, one seldom sees any such banners. Patients feel embarrassed to let even their family members and relatives know about fertility problems.

10. According to a 1994 survey in Beijing done by Edward Malinovski (personal communication), half of the respondents indicated that *zhongyi* should be consulted when a person suffers depression.

11. See Xu 1994; Young 1989.

12. My own observation in hospitals of Chinese medicine in Beijing does not support such a clear-cut distinction between patients from rural areas and cities. Patients from the rural areas and cities both present emotional symptoms. There may be some difference in verbal style. The well-educated patients may readily use more technical words such as *yayi* 压抑 (depressed) or *jiaolu* 焦虑 (anxious), while the less educated patients may simply use everyday expressions such as *xinqing buhao* 心情不好 (heart-emotion not feeling good), *xinli nanshou* 心里难受 (uncomfortable inside the heart), *faji* 发急 (worried and anxious), or *fahuo* 发火 (getting angry).

13. Lee 1996: 438.

14. Yamamoto et al. 1985

15. Zheng et al. 1986.

16. See Fabrega 1990.

17. Pollock 1996:321.

18. Jackson 1994:212.

19. Fabrega 1990:662.

20. Lee and Wang 1995:104.

21. The Chinese translation for CFS is *pilao zonghezheng* 疲劳综合症. *Zhongyi* doctors tend to relate the syndrome to such pathological conditions as "weariness" (*juan*)," "sluggishness," (*xieduo* 解堕), "sleeplessness and lack of energy" (*kunbo* 困薄), and "tired four limbs" (*sizhi buju* 四肢不举) described in *zhongyi* classics. According to *zhongyi* diagnosis, the conditions have something to do with an imbalance in functions of visceral systems caused by stagnant emotions (*qingzhi buchang* 情志不畅) over physical/mental exertions (*laoyi guodu* 劳役过度) and external pathogenic attacks (*ganshou waixie* 感受外邪).

22. See Hall and Ames (1987) for comparison of Western transcendental ontology and a Confucius immanental cosmos.

23. See Leder 1995.

24. Zito 1997:52.

25. Scheper-Hughes and Lock 1986:10.

26. See Hall and Ames 1987.

27. Good 1977:39.

28. Ames 1997:150.

29. Tung 1994:487.

30. Elvin 1993:219.

31. Ots 1994:117.

32. For lack of a better word to convey the sense of presence of the whole person including body, emotion, intellect, and spirit, I translate '*ti*' as "body personally" though it sounds awkward.

33. Brownell 1994:16.

34. Ibid.,17.

35. Brownell 1994 points out that "with the introduction of Western science and physical education, the linguistic usages of '*ti*' became much more detached, objective, and instrumental than was formerly the case" (17). To some extent, this may be true, especially in professional sports. However, to claim that in today's China, "the instrumental, gender-neutral body is unquestionably the focus of the culture of the body" is an overgeneralization.

36. The Chinese words for body-person (*shen* 身), spirit-vitality (*shen* 神), and the kidney (*shen* 肾) are homonyms. When they appear not in combination with other Chinese words, I add tones to distinguish them. Thus, *shen* as body-person will not be marked, but as spirit-vitality will be *shén* with a second tone and as kidney will be *shèn* with a fourth tone.

37. According to the dictionary of *Shouwen Jiezi* 说文解字, the original meaning of *jing* was "selected rice" (*ze mi ye* 择米也), and later the meaning was extended to anything that is the best of its kind (*fan qu hao zhi cheng* 凡取好之称).

38. Porkert (1974) translates *jing* as "structive potential."

39. *Shén* is often translated as "spirit". Porkert 1974 translates it as configurative force.

40. See Lin 198.

41. *Neijing: Suwen* (3:8). See Shangdong Yixueyuan 1982:124.

42. Li and Liu 1989:204.

43. Tung 1994:486.

44. See Ots 1994.

45. Zhong 1988:283.

46. Shandong Zhongyi Xueyuan 1982:913.

47. Farquhar 1994:26.

48. Ibid.

49. Li Y. 1995:20.

50. Desjarlais 1994:65.

51. Ibid., 68.

52. Needham 1956.

53. Sivin 1987:67.

54. Ibid., 63.

55. Shandong Zhongyi Xuyuan 1982:5.

56. Martin Schoenhals (1993:165), in his ethnographic studies of a Chinese middle school, notices that Chinese place positive value on being *huoyue* (active and energetic).

57. See Yan 1996; Yang 1994.

58. Li Y. 1995: 32.

59. Yan 1996:103.

60. *Yijing Suhui ji: Wuyu Lun* 医经溯洄集: 五郁论 (comments on medical classics: five types of yu) by Wang Andao (1332–1391) states: "Most disorders of *qi* come from *yu. Yu* by meaning is obstruction of the passage." See chapters 4 and 5 for more detailed discussions of *yu*.

61. In his *Danxi Xinfa: Liu Yu* 丹溪心法: 六郁 (methods of danxi: six types of yu), Zhu Danxi (1281–1358) claims, "When the blood and *qi* are circulating in harmony, one will not fall ill; once the circulation is stagnant, various illnesses may appear. Many illnesses result from stagnation."

62. Shweder 1985:193.

63. Kleinman 1986 maintains that "in modern times the indigenous Chinese category, *yu*, has not been widely used, in either traditional Chinese medicine or the popular culture (42)." However, my observation shows the opposite. *Yu* is a very common concept in modern *zhongyi* practice. *Yuzheng* (syndrome of stagnation), a type of *qingzhi* (emotion-mind) disorder, is a common *zhongyi* disorder.

64. Farquhar 1994:32.

65. See Lee and Wang 1995.

66. See Fabrega 1990.

67. See Lee 1996.

68. See Kleinman 1980, 1986; Ots 1990, 1994.

69. Ots 1994:119.

70. Even Confucius allowed for "excess" of emotion and justified it within certain social relations and circumstances. An instance in *Lunyu* 论语 (*The Analects* 11:10) is an interesting illustration. When his favorite student, Yan Yuan, died, Confucius was overcome with grief and cried excessively. One of his followers reminded Confucius that he went too far in his grief and that he seemed to violate what he had been teaching, namely, "moderation." Confucius replied: "I grieve with abandon [*you tong hu* 有恸乎]?; if I don't grieve with abandon for him, then for whom?" (*fei fu ren zhi wei tong er shei wei* 非夫人之恸而谁为).

71. See Potter 1988.

72. See Li Y 1995.

73. See Zhuang Chu *"Hongyang Zhonghua 'hehe wenhua' chuyi* 弘扬中华 '和合文化' 刍议 (Comments on Promoting Chinese Culture of Harmony) in *People's Daily* April 25, 1998.

74. Li Y 1995:19.

75. See Li 1995:23.

76. For detailed analysis on Chinese social exchanges, see Yan 1995; Yang 1993.

77. Li Y 1995:24.

78. The Chinese original is *"yi ta ping ta wei zhi he, gu neng feng er wu gui zhi, ruo yi tong bi tong, jin nai qi yi* 以他平他谓之和, 故能丰而物归之。若以同裨同, 尽乃弃已。"

79. Ames and Hall 1987:166.

CHAPTER IV

1. See Abu-Lughod 1988; Lutz 1987, 1988; and White, 1993.

2. See Cosdas 1990, 1993, 1994; Desjaleis 1992; Lock and Sheper-Hughes 1987; and Ots 1990, 1994.

3. See Kleinman 1980, 1986.

4. See Ots 1990, 1994.

5. Potter and Potter 1990:180–195.

6. See Kipnis 1997.

7. See Schoenhals 1993; Yan 1996.

8. Schoenhals 1993:166

9. Ibid.

10. While involved in editing a Chinese-English dictionary, I noticed that the Chinese language does not linguistically mark the distinction between what is causal and what is caused. The exact relationship has to be determined in the context. The same word out of context can mean both causal and caused. It seems the agent, the action, and the event mutually entail each other.

11. White 1993.

12. Solomon 1993:265.

13. Ames 1992:100.

14. According to Lau and Ames (1996), one is understood "in the sense that it is a continuous plenum, so that everything is related and dependent upon everything else."

15. See Xunzi: Zhengming (ca. 240 BCE). The Chinese original is *"xing zhi haowu, xi, nu, ai, le wei zhi qing* 性之好恶, 喜怒哀乐谓之情."

16. Quoted in *Hanyu Dacidian* 汉语大词典 7:576.

17. Chad Hansen 1995.

18. Solomon 1995:264.

19. See Hu 1944; Hwang 1994; King 1988; Schoenhals 1993; and Yan 1996.

20. See Hu 1944; King 1988.

21. Bond and Hwang 1986: 247.

22. King 1988.

23. Bond and Hwang 1986 classify the Chinese face behavior into six categories. These are enhancing one's own face, enhancing another's face, losing one's own face, hurting other's face, saving one's own face, and saving another's face.

24. Schoenhals 1993:70.

25. See Schoenhals 1993.

26. Hwang 1987.

27. Kleinman and Kleinman 1991:287.

28. Yan 1996.

29. Potters and Potter 1990:189.

30. Yan 1996:139.

31. Schoenhals 1993:151.

32. Lutz 1985:72.

33. *Lunyu* 论语 (*The Analects*). The Chinese original is "吾日三省吾身: 为人谋而不忠乎? 与朋友交而不信乎? 传不习乎?

34. *People's Daily*, June 6, 1998.

35. Yan 1996:122.

36. *Zhongyi* doctors usually do not make distinctions between *qing* 情 and *zhi* 志 when both refer to emotions. However, some *zhongyi* scholars argue that though both *qing* and *zhi* share the same meanings, they are different in emphasis. *Qing* is observable from outside, and *zhi* is hidden inside. See Li and Liu 1989:213. In other words, *zhi* are emotions in latency (*weifa* 未发), and *qing* are activated or demonstrated emotions. *Qiqing* (seven *qing* emotions) are regrouped in *wuzhi* (five *zhi* emotions) in order to correspond with the five visceral systems.

37. Kleinman and Kleinman 1991.

38. Sivin 1995:II–2.

39. Ots 1990:27.

40. In 1992, Deng Xiaopin on his trip in south China published his speech, which called for fundamental economic reform. Following the speech, the whole nation plunged wholeheartedly into the ocean of the market economy.

41. Li and Liu 1989:213–214.

42. *Neijing: Suwen* 2:5. The Chinese original is "人有五脏化五气, 以生喜怒悲忧恐惊."

43. The term *sanjiao* is sometimes translated as "three burners," but the actual physiological functions of *sanjiao* have nothing to do with burning. As Farhquar 1994 points out, the concept is almost impossible to translate since it is not an object and its characteristics have varied over the centuries. Based on my own observation, the concept was frequently used to refer to the three vaguely designated locations that separate internal organ systems into upper, middle, and lower fields.

44. Farquhar 1994:91.

45. Yin et al 1983:29.

46. Farqhuar 1994:94.

47. See Kuriyama 1999:25. A Chinese doctor, placing his fingers at three different positions of both wrists, reads at least 12 different pulses, which register information relating to different visceral systems.

48. Zhongyi teaches that clear and fluent speech depends on healthy heart functions, because *xin*-the heart governs *shen* (vitality, consciousness, spirit).

49. For more systematic information on the five transformative phases and the traditional Chinese medicine, see Porkert 1974 and Sivin 1988.

50. Sivin 1988:73.

51. Farquhar 1994:96.

52. The phase that produces the other phase is figuratively called "mother," and the phase that is produced is called "son." Therefore between the pair of the liver and the heart, the liver system is "the mother" and the heart is "the son."

53. The kidney is the water phase and is supposed to produce the wood phase of the liver.

54. *Neijing: Suwen* 2:5.

55. These emotion terms do not find exact corresponding meanings in English. *Si*, for example, has the meanings of "thinking," "worry," and "longing". *You* and *bei* are interchangeable here, meaning both "sorrow" and "concerns." *Kong* (fear) here also incorporates the meaning of *jing* (fright).

56. Wang and Li 1988:44.

57. See Yin et al. 1983:54–56.

58. Ibid.

CHAPTER V

1. Zhao et al. 1987. Today, *zhenghou* classification and definition remain a much debated issue, and it looks like this situation will remain for a long time to come.

2. Farquhar (1994) translates *zheng* 証 as "syndrome" for the sake of convenience. *Zheng* 証 is not an atemporal group of symptoms that collectively characterize an illness or disorder as 'syndrome' in English suggests, but a recurrent type or pattern of symptom configuration over a period of time. Any slight change in the symptom pattern may result in a reconfiguration and thus a different *zheng*. In this book, I use to translate *zheng* as a "pattern.".

3. Scheid 2002:200–237.

4. Zhao et al. 1987:7–9.

5. Zhao et al. 1987:8.

6. Farquhar 1994: 46.

7. Farquhar 1994:55–59.

8. Ibid., 58.

9. Some *zhongyi* scholars argue that *liujing bianzheng* is essentially the same as *bagang bianzheng*. See Feng et al. 2004:10–16.

10. The clear articulation of *bagang bianzheng* is traced to the Ming scholar–physician Zhang Jiebin (1562–1639). His "liang gang" 两纲 (two rubrics: yin and yang) and "*liu bian*" 六变 (six variations): *biao-li* 表里 (exterior and interior), *han-re* 寒热 (cold and hot), *xu-shi* 虚实 (deplete and replete)" include all the content of today's eight rubrics. However, to elevate *banggang bianzheng* to the position of the most important system of pattern differentiation was a more recent development in the 1950s and 60s. See Scheid 2002:200–237.

11. The illness location here should not be understood as the pathological site in an "anatomo-clinical perspective," but rather refers to "the location where *bingxie*" 病邪 (pathogenic factors) manifest. See Feng et al. 2004:12.

12. Liu 1988:231.

13. Zhao et al. 1987:4.

14. Ibid.

15. The character *yu* 郁 itself also suggests *qi* stagnation rather than blood stagnation, which is usually referred to by a different character, *yu* 瘀.

16. Farquhar 1994.

17. Ibid., 38.

18. See Farquhar 1994: chapter 4, for a detailed analysis of *zhongyi* classification.

19. Zhao et al. 1987:7.

20. In spring 1984, the first conference on *zhongyi zhenghou guifan* 中医证候规范 (standardization of *zhongyi* syndrome patterns) was held in Beijing. The specialists discussed the names, concepts, classification, and diagnostic standards of *zhenghou* (syndrome patterns). Subsequently, several influential texts on *zhenghou* standardization and diagnosis were published, such as *Zhongyi Zhenghou Zhenduan Xue* 中医证候诊断学 (The Diagnostics of *zhongyi* Syndrome Patterns) 1987 by Zhao Jinduo et al., *Zhongyi Zhenghou Bianzhi Guifan* 中医证候辨治轨范 (Standards of Differentiation and Treatment of *Zhongyi* Syndrome Patterns) 1989 by Leng Fangnan et al., and *Zhongyi Zhenghou Guifan* 中医证候规范 (Standardization of *Zhongyi* Syndrome Patterns) 1990 by Deng Tietao et al.

21. See Farquhar 1994: introduction.

22. I translate *bing* as "illness" or "disorder" to mark a distinction from the biomedical concept of "disease," which are understood as discrete biological and psychophysiological entities, resulting from lesions or abnormal functions of any structure, part, or system of an organism. The dichotomy between disease and illness has been a key concept in medical anthropology. Disease is a primary malfunction of psychobiological processes, while an illness is a secondary psychosocial experience and meaning of the primary disease. See Kleinman 1980:72. However, *bing* does not conform to such a dichotomy. It is a disorder that recognizes both psychophysiological and psychosocial dimensions.

23. Zhao et al. 1987:8.

24. Zhang et al. 1985.

25. See Feng, et al. 2004:14. Ren Yingqiu also points out that *taiyang* 太阳 (the great yang illness, one of the six cold damage illnesses) is not an independent illness but one *zhenghou* (pattern) of the cold damage illnesses. See Chen, 2003.

26. See Chen, 1997.

27. Ibid.

28. Ibid. Chen refers to this process as "*bian benzhi lunzhi*" 辨本质论治 (differentiation of roots/essence and determining therapies).

29. See Zhao, et al. 1987:2–3.

30. See Chen 1997. See also Liangchun Zhu, 2003. According to Zhu, except for very few cases, such as malaria (*nueji* 疟疾) and jaundice (*huandan* 黄疸), for most *zhongyi* illnesses, differentiation of patterns is fundamental, while the illness names are only significant as secondary references.

31. See Cheng, 2003. *Zhenghou Guifan Yanjiu de Si Da Jiaodian Wenti* 证候规范的 四大焦点问题 (Four Fundamental Issues Regarding Zhenghou Standardization). The anecdote of Professor Lu Guangshen treating AIDS in Tanzania is also an interesting illustration. In 1987, Professor Lu went to Tanzania with a team of medical specialists to help in treating the AIDS endemic in the country. He caused a considerable stir by stating that although he had never encountered a case of AIDS in China, he was confident that the disease could be treated with *zhongyi*. Again, the idea is that as long as a pattern of manifestations could be differentiated, the disease is then treatable with Chinese medicine. See Jingjing Hu, 2004 *Zhongguo Yaoshi Zhoukan* 中国药师周刊 (Chinese Pharmacists Weekly), VL. 2204.

32. The six principal patterns are *taiyang* 太阳, *yangming* 阳明, *shaoyang* 少阳, *taiyin* 太阴, *shaoyin* 少阴, and *jueyin* 厥阴.

33. See Feng and Zhang 2004:3–24. See also Scheid 2004:203–204.

34. Ren Yinqiu et al., 1986:126–131.

35. Ibid., 159–164. Although the concept and method of *bianzheng* can be found as early as in *Neijing* 内经 (The Inner Classics), the actual term "bianzheng lunzhi" or 'bianzheng shizhi' did not appear in records until the Ming and Qing period. "*Bianzheng shizhi*" first appeared in *Shenzhai Yi Shu* 慎斋遗书 (Book by Shenzhai) by the Ming physician Zhou Shenzhai (1508–1586). '*Bianzheng lunzhi*' first appeared in Yimen Banghe 医门棒喝 (1829) by the Qing physician Zhang Nan.

36. See Zhen et al. (1991:423–438). Yang Zemin (1893–1948), another scholar-physician of the time, argued that Chinese medicine emphasizes differentiation of patterns for the purpose of using drugs and Western medicine emphasizes knowing diseases for the purpose of discriminating the location of a disease. See Scheid 2002:216.

37. Several scholars of Chinese medicine mentioned an obvious relationship between the *zhongyi* diagnostics "*bianzheng lunzhi*" and the modern Chinese term for "dialectics"—*bianzhengfa* (辩证法). See Unschult 1992:52–61; Farquhar 1994; and Scheid 2002:209–214. Tian (2005) argues that "dialectics" found in the West philosophic tradition is not the same as the Chinese version of *bianzhengfa*, which draws heavily on the traditional Chinese style of thought *tongbian* (continuity through changes). In this sense, the *zhongyi* scholar-physicians' enthusiasm about *bianzhengfa* in the 1950s and

60s should be understood much more than just following "an ideologically correct" line. Rather, *bianzhengfa* offers a set of easily accessible vocabulary for scholars to articulate the *zhongyi* way of doing medicine that shares the same intellectual roots in ancient Chinese philosophical thought.

38. Scheid 2002:209–214.

39. Zhao, et al., 1987:8.

40. See also Sheid 2002:220–222.

41. Written by the Han scholar-physician Zhang Zhongjing.

42. In contemporary *zhongyi* clinics, biomedical disease names are frequently used. In fact, patients are more familiar with many common biomedical disease names than with *zhongyi* illness names. Adopting the more scientific biomedical disease classifications has been promoted by quite a few *zhongyi* physicians, including Shi Jinmo and Zhang Cigong, and other influential scholar-physicians. See Scheid 2002:221. If a pathological condition is not identified as *bentun* (running pig illness) but with a biomedical disease term, such as hysteria, the physician is directed to a different course of resources and the connection is made between the particular case and the biomedical sources. In any case, the biomedical disease name used in a *zhongyi* context does not function the same way as it does in a biomedical clinic. It does not lead to systematic matching with therapies. See Zhu 2003.

43. *Qingzhi bing* (emotion-related disorders) is also referred to as "*shenzhibing*" (mind-related disorders). Both are seen as attributable to internal injuries due to excess of the seven emotions and manifested with bodily, emotional-mental symptoms. They are interchangeable in use, though the latter is used less frequently. Li et al. (1993:59) refers to *baihe bing* 百合病 (an illness commonly listed as *qingzhi bing*) as "*shenzhi zhi bing*" 神志之病 (mind-related disorders). In the same book, the authors also state explicitly that "mind disorders are also called *qingzhi bing*" (260). Although the term *qingzhi* appears as illness factors in the earliest medical classics and the various *qingzhi*-related disorders are recorded and described as early as in *Neijing*, the actual combination of *qingzhi* and *bing* (illness, disorder) might be a more recent development.

44. Since symptoms of *dian* 癫 and *kuang* 狂 cannot be completely separate, and they often appear alternately, *dian* and *kuang* are often listed under the one disorder of *duankuang* 癫狂 (apathy and madness). See Li et al. 1993:260. The authors write "*shenzhi bing* (mind-related disorders), also called *qingzhi bing* (emotion-related disorders), include such illness as *diankuang, yuzheng* 郁证 (stagnation illness), and *bentunqi* 奔豚气 (running pig syndrome)."

45. In Li and Liu 1989, *dian* and *kuang* are listed separately from the category of *qingzhi* disorders, which include *yuzheng* (stagnation illness), *zangzao* (visceral vexation), *meiheqi* (plume pit syndrome), *baihuobing* (hundred confusions syndrome), and so on.

46. Zhang et al. eds. 1985.

CHAPTER VI

1. Li and Liu 1989:514.

2. See *Jingyue Quanshu* 景岳全书 (*The complete works of zhang jingyue*).

3. See note 6 in chapter 2 for information on *Huangdi Neijing* 黄帝内经 (*The Yellow Emperor's Internal Medicine*).

4. *Zhubing Yuanhou Lun* 诸病源候论 (*On the Origins of Various Illnesses*) was written in 610 CE by the Sui physician Chao Yuanfang and his associates.

5. *Gujin Yitong Daquan* 古今医统大全 (*Complete Collection of Principal Medical Works from Ancient Time to the Present*) was written by Ming physician Xu Chunfu (1520–1596) and published in 1556.

6. In contemporary usage, *jie* 结 refers more to the congestion that has been formed into tangible lumps, whereas *yu* 郁 is more about obstruction of flow of qi that is formless and intangible.

7. See note 4.

8. See *Danxi Xinfa: Liu Yu* 丹溪心法:六郁 (*Danxi's Healing Methods : The Six Stagnations*).

9. Ibid.

10. See *Yijing Suhui Ji* 医经溯洄集 (*Collected Reflections on the Medical Classics*) (1368).

11. See *Tuiqiu Shi Yi: Yubing* 推求师意: 郁病 (Understanding the Master's Teachings: Stagnation Illness) by Dai Sigong. This could be the earliest appearance of the term combining '*yu*' and '*bing*' in *zhongyi* texts. See Ren et al. 1984:96–102. The combination of '*yu*' and '*zheng*' did not appear until the Ming dynasty when the scholar-physician Yu Tuan first used the term in his book, *Yixue Zhengzhuan* 医学正传 (*The Orthodox History of Medicine*) (1515). See Li and Liu 1989: 103.

12. See Ren et al. 1984:118–120.

13. See *Jingyue Quanshu* 景岳全书 (*The Complete Works of Zhang Jingyue*), chapter 19.

14. Quoted in Ren at al. 1984:212–218.

15. See Ye Tianshi *Lin Zheng Zhinan Yi'an: Yuzheng* 临证指南医案: 郁证 (Guide to Clinical Practice with Medical Cases).

16. See Li and Liu 1989; Zhang et al. 1985:121–124.

17. In biomedicine, a specialist is more defined by training; however, in Chinese medicine, a *zhuanjia* (specialist) is defined mainly by his or her clinical experience and efficacy in treating certain problems.

18. See Li and Liu 1989:517.

19. Chao Yuanfang, a well-known doctor of the Yuan dynasty, uses the terms *jieqi bing* or *qi bing* (illness of congealed *qi*) to refer to the same illness manifestation type as the plum pit *qi* or *qi* stagnation illness. In fact, *qi bing* used here by the doctor has a double meaning; one is the disordered *qi* circulation in the body, and the second is the disorder caused by *qi* (anger). The patient immediately read it as the second meaning.

20. See Zhang et al. 1985:125.

21. See Li and Liu 1989.

22. See chapter 3 of this book for a discussion of *du* 度 (degree).

23. The patient's mother did not reveal any details regarding the nature of the trauma (*ciji*), and the doctor did not ask about it.

24. Zhen et al. 1991:104.

25. See Li 1993:757.

26. Cited in Li and Liu 1989:112.

27. See *Jingyue Quanshu* 景岳全书 (The Complete Works of Zhang Jingyue).

CHAPTER VII

1. Portions of this chapter appear in my article "Negotiating a path to efficacy in a clinic of traditional Chinese medicine." Forthcoming in Culture, Medicine and Psychiatry. Springer Netherlands.

2. Conversation analysis (CA), developed within the paradigm of ethnomethodology, emerged in the 1960s as a result of the pioneering works by Harvey Sacks, Gail Jefferson, Emanual Schegloff, and others. CA provides analytical resources and methodological procedures for analyzing naturally occurring human interactions. See C. Goodwin and J. Heritage 1990. Refer to appendix 1 for the transcription conventions.

3. See Atkinson and Heath 1981; Fisher and Todd 1983; Labov and Fanshel 1977; Heath 1984; Mishler 1984; Pendleton and Hasler 1983; and Tanner 1976; West 1984.

4. Labov and Fanshel 1977.

5. Hutchby & Wooffitt 1998:14.

6. Goodwin and Heritage 1990:288. See also Hutchby and Wooffitt 1998:13–17.

7. See Frankel 1983; Heath 1986.

8. See Frankel 1983; Heath 1986; Mishler 1984.

9. West 1984:34.

10. Mishler 1984:53.

11. Goodwin and Heritage 1990:283.

12. Bilmes 1992:571.

13. Mishler 1984:35.

14. For detailed analysis of *kanbing* in *zhongyi* clinics, see Judith Farquhar's book *Knowing Practice* 1994.

15. Sivin 1995:3.

16. Beijing Medical School 1975:44.

17. See Li and Liu 1989:203.

18. See Farquhar 1994.

19. In the transcript, D stands for doctor and P for patient.

20. *Jiaolu* is an introduced biomedical concept. When used in *zhongyi* context, it refers more to a vague feeling of uneasiness or restlessness, than to a psychiatric concept of "anxiety". A *zhongyi* term for the symptom might be *zuowo bu'an* 坐卧不安 (restless) or *jizao* 急躁 (anxious), or *jingzhang* 紧张 (nervous).

21. "*Uhn*" in this case is uttered with a short first tone. If it is uttered with a long, strong fourth tone, it can be understood as a confirmation.

22. Bian Que, a legendary physician from more than two thousands years ago, is well known for his examinations by looking at the patient and taking his or her pulse.

23. Bilmes 1988:165.

24. Normally, *bianzheng* (differentiate syndromes) and *lunzhi* (determine treatment) form a continuous process. There is no clear distinction between these two parts. However, it is always clear that *bianzheng* comes before *lunzhi*, and it is the basis for determining a therapy.

25. Also known as liver *qi* stagnation (*ganqi yujie* 肝气郁结) caused by blocked flow of emotions (*qingzhi bushu* 情志不舒).

26. Sometimes it goes "xiaojigengfang 效即更方" (if the effect has been achieved, change the formula).

27. Etkin 1988:302. Etkin argues that healing should be understood as a process. Efficacy might mean either an "ultimate outcome" of full symptom remission or a "proximate effect" of partial remission or some physical signs that indicate the healing is under way.

28. Kleinman 1995:33.

29. Etkin 1988:299.

30. *Guide to Clinical Practice with a Collection of the Cases* by famous Qing doctor Ye Tianshi, which was compiled by his student Hua Youyun in 1746.

31. Zhang at al. 1985:123.

32. In his article "The Angry Liver, the Anxious Heart, and the Melancholy Spleen," Ots (1990) shows that in Chinese medicine functions of the visceral systems are understood as isomorphic with the corresponding emotions.

33. As Labov and Fanshel (1977) show in their analysis of therapeutic discourse, "the therapist is an expert at interpreting the emotions of others." The therapist has the authority to judge not only the patient's interpretation of others' emotions but also her claim about her own feelings. A *zhongyi* doctor does not have that kind of authority over the patient's emotional experience. On the contrary, *zhongyi* tends to hold that one can never know exactly what another person actually experiences outside of what the other person tells you about how he or she feels. In *zhongyi* context, patients remain the authoritative voice of their own experience. A doctor's claim about a patient's experience is subject to the patient's confirmation.

34. Quoted in Zhang et al. 1985:123.

35. See *Jingyue Quanshu: Yuzheng Mo* 《景岳全书:郁证谟》 (*The Complete Works of Zhang Jingyue*: Stagnation illness) by Zhang Jiebin during the 1630s. The patronizing tone toward female patients is common in the medical classics. Women are presented as if they were children whose desires can be satisfied, but they are not capable of being enlightened. However, although not many contemporary *zhongyi* physicians disagree with Zhang about healing emotions with emotions, they do not assume his outright gendered approach to stagnant emotions. Women, active in the public sphere in contemporary China, are also counseled to be broad-minded and flexible, as shown in this case.

36. Sivin 1995:II:16.

37. Tseng et al. 1995:292.

38. See Needham 1956.
39. Arthur and Joan Kleinman 1995:153–154.
40. Farquhar 1994.
41. Hsu 1999:6.

CHAPTER VIII

1. Desjarlais 1992:249.
2. Farquhar 1992:72.
3. Kleinman 1986:43.
4. Etkin 1988:299.
5. See Farquhar 1994.

Bibliography

Abu-Lughod, Lila

1988   Veiled Sentiments: Honor and Poetry in a Bedouin Society. Berkeley: University of California Press.

Abu-Lughod, Lila, and Catherine Lutz, eds.

1989   *Language and Politics of Emotion*. Cambridge: Cambridge University Press.

Atkinson, Maxwell J., and John Heritage, eds.

1984   *Structures of Social Action: Studies in Conversation Analysis*. Cambridge: Cambridge University Press.

Ames, Roger T.

1984   The Meaning of Body in Classical Chinese Philosophy. *International Philosophical Quarterly* 24:39–54.

1991   Introduction. In *Interpreting Culture through Translation*. Roger Ames, Chan Sin-wai, and Ng Mau-Sang, eds. Hong Kong: Chinese University Press.

1992   Chinese Rationality: An Oxymoron? *Journal of Indian Council of Philosophical Research* 9 (2) 95–119.

1993   Introduction to Part Three: On Body as Ritual Practice. In *Self as Body in Asian Theory and Practice*. Thomas P. Kasulis, Wimal Dissanagake, and Roger Ames, eds. Albany: State University of New York Press.

1997   The Chinese Concept of Selfhood. In E. Deutsch & R. Bontekoe eds., *A Companion to World Philosophies*. Blackwell.

Angel, Ronald, and Peter J. Guarnaccia

1990   Mind, Body, and Culture: Somatization among Hispanics. *Social Sciences and Medicine*, 28 (12): 1229–1238.

Atkinson, P, and C. C. Heath, eds.

1981   *Medical Work: Reality and Routines*. Farnborough: Grower.

Averil, James R.

1985   The Social Construction of Emotion: With Special Reference to Love. In *Social Construction of Person*. Kenneth J. Gergen and Keith D. Davis, eds., New York: Springer-Verlag.

Becker, Joseph, and Arthur Kleinman, eds.

1991 *Psychosocial Aspects of Depression.* Hillsdale: Lawrence Erlbaum. Beijing Medical College

1975 *Zhongyi Linzheng Jichu* 中医临证基础 (The basics for diagnosis in Chinese medicine). Beijing: People's Education.

Bilmes, Jack

1985 "Why That Now?" Two Kinds of Conversational Meaning. *Discourse Processes* 8:319–355.

1986 *Discourse and Behavior.* New York: Plenum.

1988 The Concept of Preference in Conversation Analysis. *Language in Society* 17:161–181.

1992 Dividing the Rice: A Microanalysis of the Mediator's Role in a Northern Thai Negotiation. *Language in Society* 21:569–602.

Blacking, John

1977 *The Anthropology of the Body.* London: Academic.

Blake, Fred

1994 Foot-Binding in Neo-Confucian China. *Signs* 19(3): 676–712.

Blumhagen, D.

1980 Hypertension: A Folk Illness with a Medical Name. *Culture, Medicine and Psychiatry* 4:197–228.

Bond, Michael Harris, ed.

1986 *The Psychology of the Chinese People.* Oxford: Oxford University Press.

Bond, Michael Harris, and Kwang-kuo Hwang

1986 The Social Psychology of Chinese People. In *The Psychology of the Chinese People.* Michael H. Bond, ed. Pp. 213–264. Oxford: Oxford University Press.

Bowers, John Z., J. William Hess, and Nathan Sivin, eds.

1987 *Science and Medicine in Twentieth-Century China: Research and Education.* Ann Arbor: Center for Chinese Studies, the University of Michigan.

Brownell, Susan

1995 *Training the Body for China.* Chicago: University of Chicago Press.

Browner, C. H., B. R. Ortiz de Montellano, and A. J. Rubel

1988 A Methodology for Cross-Cultural Ethnomedical Research. *Current Anthropology* 29 (5):681–701.

Cai, Jingfeng

1988 Integration of Traditional Chinese Medicine with Western Medicine—Right or Wrong? *Social Science and Medicine* 27(5): 521–529.

Calhoun, Craig, Edward LiPuma, and Moishe Postone, eds.

1993 *Bourdieu: Critical Perspectives.* Chicago: University of Chicago Press.

Chen, Xiaoye

1997 *Lun Zhongyi Binglixue Zheng, Bing Gainian de Tongyi* 论中医病理学证, 病概念的同一 (The monistic explanation of zheng and bing in zhongyi pathology). Journal of Traditional Chinese Medicine. (8):499.

Cheng, Dongqi

2003   *Zhenghou Guifan Yanjiu de Si Da Jiaodian Wenti* 证候规范研究的四大焦点问题 (The four focal problems with standardization of patterns of syndromes). http://www.cntcm.com .cn/text/1880-b.htm, accessed May 19.

Cheng, Tai-Ann

1995   Neuroses in Taiwan: Findings from a Community Survey. In *Chinese Society and Mental Health*. T. Y. Lin, W. S. Tseng, and E. K. Yeh, eds. Pp.167–180. Hong Kong: Oxford University Press.

Cheung, Fanny M.

1982   Psychological Symptoms among Chinese in Urban Hong Kong. *Social Science and Medicine* 16: 1339–1344.

1987   Psychopathology among Chinese People. In *The Psychology of the Chinese People*. M. H. Bond, ed. Pp. 171–212. Hong Kong: Oxford University Press.

1989   The Indigenization of Neurasthenia in Hong Kong. *Culture, Medicine and Psychiatry* 13:227–241.

1995   Facts and Myths about Somatization among the Chinese. In *Chinese Societies and Mental Health*. T. Y. Lin et al, eds. Pp.156–166. Hong Kong: Oxford University Press.

Chu, Zhuang

1998   Hongyang Zhonghua "Hehe Wenhua" Chuyi 弘扬中华 "合和文化" 刍议. (Thoughts on promoting Chinese "culture of harmony"). *People's Daily*, April 15.

Cicourel, Aaron

1993   Aspects of Structural and Processual Theories of Knowledge. In *Bourdieu: Critical Perspectives*. Craig Calhoun, Edward LiPuma,. and Moishe Postone, eds. Pp. 89–115. Chicago: University of Chicago Press.

Cohen, A.

1992   Prognosis for Schizophrenia in the Third World: A Reevaluation of Cross-Cultural Research. *Culture, Medicine and Psychiatry* 16(1): 53–75.

Cooper, J. E, and N. A. Sartorius

1977   Cultural and Temporal Variations in Schizophrenia: A Speculation on the Importance of Industrialization. *British Journal Psychiatry* 130:50–55.

Csordas, Thomas J.

1988   Elements of Charismatic Persuasion and Healing. *Medical Anthropology Quarterly* 2:121–142.

1990   Embodiment as a Paradigm for Anthropology. *Ethos* 18:5–47.

1993   Somatic Modes of Attention. *Cultural Anthropology* 8(2):135–156.

1994   *Embodiment and Experience*. Cambridge: Cambridge University Press.

Csordas, Thomas, and Arthur Kleinman

1996   Therapeutic Process. In *Medical Anthropology: A Handbook of Theory and Methods*. T. Johnson and C. Sargent, eds. Pp. 3–21. Second Edition. New York: Greenwood.

Davis, Scott

1996   The Cosmobiological Balance of the Emotional and Spiritual Worlds: Phenomenological Structuralism in Traditional Chinese Medical Thought. In *Culture, Medicine and Psychiatry* 20: 83–123.

Desjarlais, Robert

1992   *Body and Emotion: The Aesthetics of Illness and Healing in the Nepal Himalayas.* Philadelphia: University of Pennsylvania Press.

Douglas, Mary

1975   *Implicit Meanings: Essays in Anthropology.* London: Routledge and Kegan Paul.
1982   *Natural Symbols: Explorations in Cosmology.* New York: Pantheon Books.

Eisenberg, David

1985   *Encounters with Qi: Exploring Chinese Medicine.* New York: Norton.

Ekman, Paul, ed.

1973   *Darwin and Facial Expression.* New York: Academic.
1980   *Face of Man: Universal Expression in a New Guinea Village.* New York: Garland.

Ekman, P., and H. Oster

1978   Facial Expressions of Emotion. *Annual Review of Psychology,* 30:517–554.

Elvin, Mark

1993   Tales of *Shen* and *Xin*: Body-Person and Heart-Mind in China during the Last 150 Years. In *Self as Body in Asian Theory and Practice.* Thomas P. Kasulis, Wimal Dissanagake, and Roger Ames, eds. Pp. 213–294. Albany: State University of New York Press.

Etkin, Nina

1988   Cultural Constructions of Efficacy. In *The Context of Medicines in Developing Countries.* S.vand der Geest and S. R. Whyte, eds. Pp. 299–326. Kluwer.
1992   "Side Effects": Cultural Constructions and Reinterpretations of Western Pharmaceuticals. *Medical Anthropology Quarterly* 6(2):99–113.

Fabrega, Horacio, Jr.

1990   The Concept of Somatization as a Cultural and Historical Product of Western Medicine. *Psychosomatic Medicine* 52:653–672.

Farquhar, Judith

1987   Problems of Knowledge in Contemporary Chinese Medical Discourse. *Social Sciences and Medicine* 24 (12):1013–1021.
1992   Time and Text: Approaching Chinese Medical Practice through Analysis of a Published Case. In *Paths to Asian Medical Knowledge.* Charles Leslie and Allan Young, eds. Pp. 62–73. Berkeley: University of California Press.
1994   *Knowing Practice: The Clinical Encounter of Chinese Medicine.* Boulder: Westview.
2002   *Appetites: Food and Sex in Post-Socialist China.* Durham and London: Duke University Press.

Featherstone, Mike, Mike Hepworth, and Bryan S. Turner

1991 *Body: Social Process and Cultural Theory.* London: Sage.

Feng, Shilun, and Zhang Chang'en

2004   *Zhang Zhongjing Yongfang Jiexi* 张仲景用方解析 (Explaining analyzing the use of formulas by Zhang Zhongjing). Beijing: People's Military Medical Press.

Fisher, S, and A. D. Todd

1983   *The Social Organization of Doctor-Patient Communication.* Washington: Center for Applied Linguistics.

Foucault, Michel
1994 *The Birth of the Clinic: An Archaeology of Medical Perception.* A. M. Sheidan Smith, trans. New York: Vintage Books.

Frake, C. O.
1961 The Diagnosis of Disease among the Subanun of Mindanao. *American Anthropology* 63:112–132.

Frank, Arthur W.
1990 Bringing Bodies Back In: A Decade Review. *Theory, Culture and Society* 7:131–162.

Frankel, R. M.
1983 The Laying on of Hands: Aspects of the Organization of Gaze, Touch, and Talk in Medical Encounter. In S. Fisher and A. D. Todd, eds., *The Social Organization of DoctorPpatient Communication.* Washington, DC: Center for Applied Linguistics.

Freund, Peter E. S.
1990 The Expressive Body: A Common Ground for the Sociology of Emotions and Health and Illness. *Sociology of Health and Illness* 12:452–457.

Furth, Charlotte, and Ch'en Shu-Yueh
1991 Chinese Medicine and the Anthropology of Menstruation in Contemporary Taiwan. *Medical Anthropology Quarterly* (6) 1:27–48.

Gergen, Kenneth
1990 Social Understanding and the Inscription of Self. In *Cultural Psychology: Essays on Comparative Human Development.* J. W. Stigler, R. A. Shweder, and G. H. Herdt, eds. Cambridge: Cambridge University Press.

Gilboa, Eva and William Revelle
1994 Personality and the Structure of Affective Responses. In *Emotions: Essays on Emotion Theory.* Stephanie H. M. van Goodzen et al., eds. Pp. 135–159. Hillsdale, New Jersey Erlbaum.

Good, B. J., and A. Kleinman
1985 Culture and Anxiety: Cross-cultural Evidence of Patterning of Anxiety Disorders. In *Anxiety and Anxiety Disorders.* A. H. Tuma and J. Maser, eds. Hillsdale: Erlbaum.

Good, Byron
1977 The Heart of What's Matter: The Semantics of Illness in Iran. *Culture, Medicine and Psychiatry* 1:25–58.
1992 Culture and Psychopathology: Directions for Psychiatric Anthropology. In *New Directions in Psychological Anthropology.* Theodore Schwartz et al., eds. Cambridge: Cambridge University Press.
1994 *Medicine, Rationality, and Experience: An Anthropological Perspective.* New York: Cambridge University Press.

Good, Byron, and M. J. Good

1980   The Meaning of Symptoms: A Cultural Hermeneutic Model for Clinical Prac-
        tice. In *The Relevance of Social Science for Medicine*. L. Eisengberg and A. Klein-
        man, eds. Pp. 165–196.

1981   The Semantics of Medical Discourse. In *Sociology of the Sciences*. E. Mendelson
        and Y. Elkana, eds. Pp. 177–212. Holland: Reidel.

1982   Toward a Meaning-centered Analysis of Popular Illness Categories: "Fright Ill-
        ness" and "Heart Distress." In *Cultural Conceptions of Mental Health and Therapy*.
        A. Marsella and G. White, eds. Pp. 141–166. Holland: Reidel.

Goodwin, Charles, and John Heritage

1990   Conversation Analysis. *Annual Review of Anthropology* 19:283–307.

Gordon, Deborah

1990   Embodying Illness, Embodying Cancer. *Culture, Medicine and Psychiatry* 14:
        275–97.

Gray, Jeffrey A.

1977   Framework for a Taxonomy of Psychiatric Disorder. In *Emotions: Essays on
        Emotion Theory*. Stephanie H. M. van Goozen et al., eds. Pp. 29–59. Hillsdale,
        New Jersey: Erlbaum.

Hall, David, and Roger T. Ames

1987   *Thinking through Confucius*. Albany: State University of New York Press.

Hanks, William F.

1993   Notes on Semantics in Linguistic Practice. In *Bourdieu: Critical Perspectives*.
        Craig Calhoun et al. eds. Pp. 139–155. Chicago: University of Chicago Press.

Hanyu Dacidian Chubanshe

1996   *Hanyu Dacidian* 汉语大词典 (Comprehensive Chinese Dictionary). Shanghai:
        Hanyu Dacidian Chubanshe.

Heath, Christian

1984   *Body Movement and Speech in Medical Interaction*. Cambridge: Cambridge Uni-
        versity Press.

Heesacker, Martin, and Margret M. Bradley

1997   Beyond Feelings: Psychotherapy and Emotion. *The Counseling Psychologist* 25
        (2):201–219.

Helman, Cecil

1984   Psyche, Soma and Society: The Social Construction of Psychosomatic Disor-
        ders. *Culture, Medicine and Psychiatry* 9 (1): 1–26.

Herzlich, Claudine, and Janine Pierret

1987   *Illness and Self in Society*. Baltimore: Johns Hopkins University Press.

Hevic, James L.

1994   Sovereignty and Subject: Constituting Relations of Power in Qing Guest Rit-
        ual. In *Body, Subject and Power in China*. Angela Zito and Tani E. Barlow, eds.
        Pp 181–200. Chicago: University of Chicago Press.

Hoizey, Dominique, and Marie-Joseph Hoizey
1993   *A History of Chinese Medicine*. Paul Bailey, trans. Vancouver: UBC.

Hsu, Elisabeth
1999   *The Transmission of Chinese Medicine*. Cambridge: Cambridge University Press.

Hsu, Jing
1995   Family Therapy for the Chinese: Problems and Strategies. In *Chinese Societies and Mental Health*. Tsung-yi Lin, Wen-shing Tseng, and Eng-Kung Yeh, eds. Hong Kong: Oxford University Press.

Hu Hsien-chin
1944   The Chinese Concept of Face. *American Anthropologist* 46: 45–66.

Hutchby, Ian, and Robin Wooffitt.
1998   *Conversation Analysis: Principles, Practices and Applications*. Cambridge: Polity.

Hwang, Kwang-kuo
1987   Face and Favor: The Chinese Power Game. *American Journal of Sociology* 92 (4): 944–974.

Jackson, Jean
1994   Chronic Pain and the Tension between the Body as Subject and Object. In *Embodiment and Experience*. Thomas Csordas, ed. Pp. 201–224. Cambridge: Cambridge University Press.

Jackson, Michael
1989   *Paths toward a Clearing: Radical Empiricism and Ethnographic Inquiry*. Blooming: Indiana University Press.

Jenkins, Janis. H.
1988   Ethnopsychiatric Interpretations of Schizophrenic Illness: The Problem of Nervios within Mexican-American Families. *Culture, Medicine and Psychiatry* 12:301–330.
1990   Culture, Emotion, and Psychiatric Disorder." In *Medical Anthropology: Contemporary Theory and Method*. C. F. Sargent and T. M. Johnson, eds. Pp. 71–87. New York: Greenwood.

Jenkins, Janis H., Arthur Kleinman, and Byron J. Good
1991   Cross-cultural Studies of Depression. In *Psychosocial Aspects of Depression*. Joseph Baker and Arthur Kleinman, eds. Pp. 67–99. Hillsdale: Erlbaum.

Jenkins, Janis H., and Martha Valiente
1994   Bodily Transactions of the Passion: *El Clor* among Salvadoran Women Refugees. In *Embodiment and Experience*. Thomas J. Csordas, ed. Pp. 163–177. Cambridge: Cambridge University Press.

Johnson, Mark
1987   *The Body in the Mind: The Bodily Basis of Meaning, Imagination, and Reason*. Chicago: University of Chicago Press.

Kasulis, Thomas P. et al., eds.
1993   *Self as Body in Asian Theory and Practice*. Albany: State University of New York Press.

King, Ambrose Y. C.

1988   Face, Shame, and Analysis of Behavior of the Chinese. In *Zhongguoren de Xinli* 中国人的心理 (The psychology of the Chinese). Guo Shuyang, ed. Taipei, Taiwan: Guiguan.

Kipnis, Andrew

1997   *Producing Guanxi: Sentiment, Self, and Subculture in a North China Village.* Durham, NC: Duke University Press.

Kirmayer, Laurence J.

1992   The Body's Insistence on Meaning: Metaphor as Presentation and Representation in Illness Experience. *Medical Anthropology Quaterly* 6 (4): 322–346.

Kitayama, S., and Markus, H. R.

1994   Introduction to Cultural Psychology and Emotion Research. In *Emotion and Culture: Empirical Studies of Mutual Influence.* S. Kitayama and H. R. Markus, eds. Pp. 1–19. Washington, DC: American Psychological Association.

Kleinman, Arthur

1980   *Patients and Healers in the Context of Culture.* Berkeley: University of California Press.

1982   Neurasthenia and Depression: A Study of Socialization and Culture in China. *Culture, Medicine and Psychiatry* 117–190.

1986   *Social Origins of Distress and Disease: Depression, Neurasthenia, and Pain in Modern China.* New Haven: Yale University Press.

1988   *The Illness Narratives: Suffering, Healing, and Human Condition.* New York: Basic Book.

Kleinman, Arthur, and Byron Good

1985   *Culture and Depression.* Berkeley: University of California Press.

Kleinman, Arthur, and Joan Kleinman

1985   Somatization: The Interconnections in Chinese Society among Culture, Depressive Experiences, and the Meaning of Pain. In *Culture and Depression.* A. Kleinman and B. Good, eds. Pp. 429–490. Berkeley: University of California Press.

1991   Suffering and Its Professional Transformation: Toward an Ethnography of Interpersonal Experience. *Culture, Medicine and Psychiatry* (5)3: 275–301.

1995   Remembering the Cultural Revolution: Alienating Pains and the Pain of Alienation/Transformation. In *Chinese Societies and Mental Health.* T. Y Lin, W. S. Tseng, and E. K. Yeh, eds. Pp. 141–155. Hong Kong: Oxford University Press.

Kleinman, Arthur, and David Mechanic

1981   Mental Illness and Psychosocial Aspect of Medical Problems in China. In *Normal and Abnormal Behavior in Chinese Culture.* A. Kleinman and Tsung-yi Lin, eds. Pp. 331–356. Dordrecht: Reidel.

Kleinman, Arthur, and Tsung-yi Lin

1981   *Normal and Abnormal Behavior in Chinese Culture.* Dordrecht: Reidel.

Kraepelin, Emil
1974 [1904] Comparative Psychiatry. In *Themes and Variations in European Psychiatry: An Anthology*. S. R. Hirsch and M. Shepherd, eds. Pp. 3–6. Bristol: Wright and Sons.

Kuriyama, Shigehisa
1999 *The Expressiveness of the Body and the Divergence of Greek and Chinese Medicine*. New York: Zone Books.

Labov, William, and David Fanshel
1977 *Therapeutic Discourse: Psychotherapy as Conversation*. New York: Academic.

Lademan, Carol, and Marina Roiseman, eds.
1996 *The Performance of Healing*. New York: Routledge.

Lakoff, George
1987 *Women, Fire, and Dangerous Things: What Categories Reveal about the Mind*. Chicago: University of Chicago Press.

Lakoff, George and Zoltan Kövecses
1987 The Cognitive Model of Anger Inherent in American English. In *Cultural Models in Language and Thought*. Naomi Quinn and Dorothy Holland, eds. Pp. 195–221. Cambridge: Cambridge University Press.

Langer, Monika M.
1989 *Merleau-Ponty's Phenomenology of Perception*. Tallahassee: Florida State University Press.

Lau, D.C. and R. T. Ames
1996 Introduction. In *Sun Pin: The Art of Warfare*. D.C. Lau and R. T. Ames, trans. New York: Ballantine Books.

Leder, Drew
1990 *The Absent Body*. Chicago: University of Chicago.

Lee, Sing
1994 The Vicissitudes of Neurasthenia in Chinese Societies: Where Will It Go from the ICD-10. *Transcultural Psychiatric Research Review* 31: 153–172.
1996 Cultures in Psychiatric Nosology: The CCMD-2-R and International Classification of Mental Disorders. *Culture, Medicine and Psychiatry* 20:421–472.

Lee, Sing, and Kit Ching Wang
1995 Rethinking Neurasthenia: The Illness Concepts of Shenjing Shuairuo among Chinese Undergraduates in Hong Kong. *Culture, Medicine and Psychiatry* 19:91–111.

Leff, Julian P.
1981 *Psychiatry around the Globe: A Transcultural View*. New York: Dekker.

Levy, R. I.
1984 Emotion, Knowing, and Culture. In *Culture Theory: Essays in Mind, Self, and Emotion*. R. A. Shweder and R. A LeVine, eds. New York: Cambridge University Press.

Li, Mucai

1987 *Huashuo Zhongyi* 话说中医 (Talking about traditional Chinese medicine). Beijing: Kexue Puji Chubanshe.

Li, Qingfu, and Liu Duzhou

1989 *Zhongyi Jingshen Bing Xue* 中医精神病学 (Zhongyi psychiatry). Tianjing: Tianjing Kexue Jishu Chubanshe.

Li, Wenrui, with Li Chi and Li Yue

1993 *Jinkui Yaolue Tangzheng Lunzhi* 金匮要略汤证论治 (On Synopsis of Golden Cabinet: Application and Comments). Beijing: Zhongguo Kexue Jishu Chubanshe.

Li, Yiyuan

1995 The Traditional Chinese Cosmology and the Behavior of Modern Enterprises. In *Zhongguo Ren de Guannian He Xingwei* 中国人的观念和行为 (The values and behavior of Chinese people). Chao Jian and Pan Naigu, eds. Pp. 17–39. Tianjing: Tianjing Renmin Chubanshe.

Liao, Yuqun

2005 *Zhongyi bu jiao 'kexue' weichang bu ke* 中医不叫科学未尝不可 (Chinese medicine doesn't have to be labeled as 'science'). In *Zhe Yan Kan Zhongyi* 哲眼看中医 (Chinese medicine through perspectives of philosophy). Zhongguo Zhongyiyao Baoshe ed. Pp. 87–94. Bejing: Kexue Jishu Chubanshe.

Lin, Keh-min

1981 Traditional Chinese Medical Beliefs and Their Relevance for Mental Illness and Psychiatry. In *Normal and Abnormal Behaviors in Chinese Culture*. A. Kleinman and T. Y. Lin, eds. Dordrecht, the Netherlands: Reidel.

Lin, Tsung-yi

1983 Psychiatry and Chinese Culture. *The Western Journal of Medicine* 139:862–867.

Lin, Tsung-yi, and Leon Eisenberg, eds.

1985 *Mental Health Planning for One Billion People*. Vancouver: University of British Columbia Press.

Liu, Yanchi

1988 *The Essential Book of Traditional Chinese Medicine*. Fang Tingyu and Chen Laidi, trans. New York: Columbia University Press.

Lock, Margaret

1993 Cultivating the Body: Anthropology and Epistemologies of Bodily Practice and Knowledge. *Annual Reviews of Anthropology* 22:133–155.

Lock, Margaret, and Pamela Dunk

1992 My Nerves Are Broken. In *Health in Canadian Society: Sociological Perspectives*. D. Coburn, C. D'Arcy, G. Torrance, and P. New, eds. Pp. 2995–3013. Toronto: Fithenry and Wimbleside.

Lock, Margaret, and Nancy Sheper-Huges

1990 A Critical-Interpretive Approach in Medical Anthropology: Rituals and Routines of Discipline and Dissent. In *Medical Anthropology*. Pp. 47–72. T. M. Johnson and C. Sargent, eds. New York: Greenwood.

Low, Setha M.

1994   Embodied Metaphors: Nerves as Lived Experience. In *Embodiment and Experience: the Existential Ground of Culture and Self*. Thomas J. Csordas, ed. Pp. 139–162. Cambridge: Cambridge University Press.

Lu, Zhaolin

1987   *Jing, Qi, Shen* 精, 气, 神. Beijing: Kexue Puji Chubanshe.

Lucas, Rodney H., and Robert J. Barrett

1995   Interpreting Culture and Psychopathology: Primitivist Themes in Cross-Cultural Debate. *Culture, Medicine and Psychiatry* 19: 287–326.

Lutz, Catherine A.

1983   Depression and the Translation of Emotional Worlds. In *Culture and Depression*. A. Kleinman and B. Good, eds. Pp. 63–100 Berkeley: University of California Press.

1988   *Unnatural Emotions: Everyday Sentiments on a Micronesian Atoll*. Chicago: University of Chicago Press.

Lutz, Catherine A., and Lila Abu-Lughod, eds.

1990   *Language and the Politics of Emotion*. Cambridge: Cambridge University Press.

Lutz, Catherine A., and Geoffrey White

1986   The Anthropology of Emotions. *Annual Review of Anthropology* 15:405–436.

Markus, H. R., and S. Kitayama.

1994   The Cultural Construction of Self and Emotion: Implications for Social Behavior. In *Emotion and Culture: Empirical Studies of Mutual Influence*. S. Kitayama and H. R. Markus, eds. Pp. 89–130.

Marsella, Anthony, and Geoffrey White, eds.

1984   *Cultural Conceptions of Mental Health and Therapy*. Boston: Reidel.

Marsella, Anthony, George DeVos, and Francis Hsu, eds.

1985   *Culture and Self: Asian and Western Perspectives*. New York: Tavistock.

Martin, Emily

1992   The End of the Body? *American Anthropologist* 19: 121–40.

Merleau-Ponty, Maurice

1986   *The Phenomenology of Perception*. Colin Smith, trans. London: Routledge and Kegan Paul.

Mishler, Elliot G.

1984   *The Discourse of Medicine: Dialectics of Medical Interviews*. Norwood: Ablex.

Moreman, Michael

1988   *Talking Culture: Ethnography and Conversation Analysis*. Philadelphia: Universtiy of Pennsylvania Press.

1991   Studying Gestures in Social Context. In *Culture Embodied*. M. Moreman & Nomura, eds. Osaka: National Museum of Ethnology.

Murphy, H. B. M., and A. C. Raman

1971   The Chronicity of Schizophrenia in Indigenous Tropical Peoples: Result of a Twelve-Year Follow-Up Survey in Mauritius. *British Journal of Psychiatry* 118:489–497.

Murphy, H. B. M., and B. M. Taumoepeau
1980   Traditionalism and Mental Health in the South Pacific: A Reexamination of an
        Old Hypothesis. *Psychological Medicine* 10:471–482.

Needham, Joseph
1956   *Science and Civilization in China*. Vols. 1 and 2. Cambridge: Cambridge Univer-
        sity Press.

Nichter, Mark
1981   Idioms of Distress: Alternatives in Expression of Psychiatry. *Culture, Medicine
        and Psychiatry* (5) 4: 379–408.

Ots, Thomas
1990   The Angry Liver, the Anxious Heart, and the Melancholy Spleen: The Phe-
        nomenology of Perceptions in Chinese Culture. *Culture, Medicine and Psychia-
        try* 14: 21–58.
1994   The Silenced Body—the Expressed Leib: On the Dialectic of Mind and Life
        in Chinese Cathartic Healing. In *Embodiment and Experience*. Thomas Csordas,
        ed. Pp. 116–138. Cambridge: Cambridge University Press.

Pedleton, D., and J. Hasler, eds.
1983   *Doctor-Patient Communication*. London: Academic.

Pollock, Donald
1996   Personhood and Illness among the Kulina. *Medical Anthropology Quarterly*
        10(3): 319–341.

Porkert, Manfred
1974   *Theoretical Foundations of Chinese Medicine: Systems of Correspondence*. Cam-
        bridge: MIT Press.

Potter, Sulamith
1988   The Cultural Construction of Emotion in Rural Chinese Social Life. *Ethos*
        16:181–208.

Potter, Sulamith Heins, and Jack M. Potter
1990   *China's Peasants: The Anthropology of a Revolution*. Cambridge: Cambridge Uni-
        versity Press.

Prince, Raymond, and Francoise Tcheng-Laroche
1987   Culture-Bound Syndromes and International Disease Classifications. *Culture,
        Medicine and Psychiatry* 2:13–19.

Psathas, George
1990   The Organization of Talk, Gaze, and Activity in a Medical Interview. In *Inter-
        action Competence*. Geoge Psathas, ed. Washington, D.C.: International Insti-
        tute for Ethnomethodology and Conversation Analysis and University Press of
        America.

Quinn, Naomi, and Dorothy Holland, eds.
1987   *Cultural Models in Language and Thought*. Cambridge: Cambridge University
        Press.

Ren, Yingqiu, Qiu Peiran, and Ding Guangdi, eds.
1994   *Zhongyi Gejia Xueshuo* 中医各家学说 (Schools of zhongyi theories). Shanghai: Shanghai Kexue Jishu Chubanshe.

Scarry, Elaine
1985   *The Body in Pain: The Making and Un-Making of the World.* New York: Oxford University Press.

Scheid, Volker
2002   *Chinese Medicine in Contemporary China: Plurality and Synthesis.* Durham and London: Duke University Press.

Scheper-Hughes, Nancy
1988   The Madness of Hunger: Sickness, Delirium, and Human Needs. *Culture, Medicine and Psychiatry* 12:429–458.
1992   Hungry Bodies, Medicine, and the State: Toward a Critical Psychological Anthropology. In *New Direction in Psychological Anthropology.* T. Schwartz, G. White, and C. Lutz, eds. Pp. 221–247. Cambridge: Cambridge University Press.

Scheper-Hughes, Nancy, and Margaret Lock
1987   The Mindful Body: A Prolegomenon to Future Work in Medical Anthropology. *Medical Anthropology Quarterly* 1(1):6–41.

Scherer, Klaus R., and Paul Ekman, eds.
1989   *Approaches to Emotion.* Hillsdale: Erlbaum.

Schoenhals, Martin
1993   *The Paradox of Power in a People's Republic of China Middle School.* Armonk: Sharpe.

Shandong Zhongyi Xueyuan and Hebei Zhongyi Xueyuan
1982   *Huangdi Neijing Suwen Jiaoshi* 黄帝内经素问校释 (Collation and comments on *Yellow Emperior's Inner Classics: Plain Questions*). Beijing: Renmin Weisheng Chubanshe.

Shen, Yu-Cun, and Wang Yu-Feng
1995   Behaviour Problems of Schoolchildren in Beijing: A Study of Prevalence and Risk Factors. In *Chinese Societies and Mental Health.* T.Y. Lin et al., eds. Pp. 57–66. Hong Kong: Oxford University Press.

Shweder, Richard
1985   Menstrual Pollution, Soul Loss, and the Comparative Study of Emotions. In *Culture and Depression: Studies in Anthropology and Cross-Cultural Psychiatry of Affect and Disorder.* A. Kleinman and B. Good, eds. Pp. 182–215. Berkeley: University of California Press.
1991   Rethinking Culture and Personality Theory. In *Thinking through Culture.* R. Shweder, ed. Cambridge: Harvard University Press.

Sivin, Nathan
1987   *Traditional Medicine in Contemporary China.* Ann Arbor: University of Michigan Press.

1995   *Medicine, Philosophy and Religion in Ancient China.* Variorum: Variorum Collected Studies Series.

Solomon, Robert C.

1993   The Cross-cultural Comparison of Emotion. In *Emotion in Asian Thoughts.* Loel Marks and Roger T. Ames, eds. Pp. 253–318. Albany: State University of New York

Tan, Eng-Seong

1981   Culture-Bound Syndromes among Overseas Chinese. In *Normal and Abnormal Behavior in Chinese Culture.* A. Kleinman and T. Y. Lin, eds. Pp. 371–386. Dordrecht: Reidel.

Tanner, B., ed.

1976   *Language and Communication in General Practice.* London: Hodder and Stoughton.

Taussig, Michael

1980   Reification and the Consciousness of the Patient. *Social Science and Medicine* 14:3–31.

Tseng, Wen-Shing

1974   The Development of Psychiatric Concepts in Traditional Chinese Medicine. *Archives of General Psychiatry* 29:569–575.

1975   The Nature of Somatic Complaints among Psychiatric Patients: The Chinese Case. *Comprehensive Psychiatry* 16: 237–245.

1995   Psychotherapy for the Chinese: Cultural Considerations. In *Chinese Societies and Mental Health.* Tsung-yi Lin, Wen-shing Tseng, and Eng-Kung Yeh, eds. Pp. 281–294. Hong Kong: Oxford University Press.

Tseng, Wen-Shing, and David Wu, eds.

1985   *Chinese Culture and Mental Health.* Orlando: Academic.

Tu, Wei-ming

1985   Selfhood and Otherness in Confucian Thought. In A. Marsella, G. DeVos, and F. Hsu, eds. *Culture and Self: Asian and Western Perspectives.* New York: Tavistock.

Tung, May P. M.

1994   Symbolic Meanings of the Body in Chinese Culture and "Somatization." *Culture, Medicine and Psychiatry* 18: 483–492.

Turner, Bryan S. et al., eds.

1991   *The Body: Social Process and Cultural Theory.* London: Sage.

Unschuld, Paul U.

1985   *Medicine in China: A History of Ideas.* Berkeley: University of California Press.

1992   Epistemological Issues and Changing Legitimation: Traditional Chinese Medicine in the Twentieth Century. In *Paths to Asian Medical Knowledge.* C. Leslie and A. Young, eds. Berkeley: University of California Press.

Veith, Ilza, trans.
1972   *The Yellow Emperor's Internal Medicine: Plain Questions*. Berkeley: University of
        California Press.

Waitzkin, Howard
1983   *The Second Sickness: Contradictions of Capitalist Health Care*. New York: Free
        Press.
1989   A Critical Theory of Medical Discourse: Text, Context, and the Structure of
        Medical Encounters. *Health and Social Behavior* 30:220–239.

Wang, Hongtu, and Li Kangzhuang
1987   *Xin 心* (Heart-mind). Beijing: Kexue Puji Chubanshe.

Ware, Norma C., and Mitchell G. Weiss
1994   Overview: Neurasthenia and the Social Construction of Psychiatric Knowl-
        edge. *Transcultural Psychiatric Research Review* 33: 101–123.

Warner, R.
1983   Recovery from Schizophrenia in the Third World. *Psychiatry* 46:197–212.
1985   *Recovery from Schizophrenia: Psychiatry and Political Economy*. London: Rout-
        ledge and Kegan Paul.

Watson-Gegeo, Karen A. and Geoffrey White, eds.
1990   *Disentangling: Conflict Discourse in Pacific Societies*. Standford: Stanford Univer-
        sity Press.

Waxler, N. E.
1979   Is Outcome for Schizophrenia Better in Nonindustrial Societies? The Case of
        Sri Lanka. *Journal of Nervous and Mental Disease* 167(3): 144–158.

Waxler-Morrison, Nancy
1992   Commentary on Cohen Prognosis for Schizophrenia in the Third World. *Cul-
        ture, Medicine and Psychiatry* 16:77–80.

West, Candace
1984   *Routine Complications*. Bloomington: Indiana University Press.

White, Geoffrey
1981   The Role of Cultural Explanations in "Somatization" and "Psychologization."
        Social Science and Medicine 16: 1519–1530.
1990a   Moral Discourse and the Rhetoric of Emotions. In *Language and the Politics of
        Emotion*. Catherine A. Lutz and Lila Abu-Lughod, eds. Pp. 46–68. Cambridge:
        Cambridge University Press.
1990b   Emotion Talk and Social Inference: Disentangling in a Solomon Islands Soci-
        ety. In *Disentangling: Conflict Discourse in Pacific Societies*. K. Watson-Gegeo and
        G. M. White, eds. Stanford: Stanford University Press.
1992   Ethnopsychology. In *New Direction in Psychological Anthropology*. G. White and
        C. Lutz, eds. Cambridge: Cambridge University Press.
1993   Emotions Inside Out: The Anthropology of Affects. In *Handbook of Emotions*.
        M. Lewis and J. M. Haviland-Jones, eds. New York: Guilford Press.

White, Geoffrey, and John Kirkpatrick, eds.

1987 *Person, Self and Experience: Exploring Pacific Ethnopsychologies.* Berkeley: University of California Press.

White, Geoffrey, and Catherine Lutz, eds.

1992 *New Direction in Psychological Anthropology.* Cambridge: Cambridge University Press.

Wierzbicka, Anna

1994 Emotion, Language, and Cultural Scripts. In *Emotion and Culture: Empirical Studies of Mutual Influence.* Shinobu Kitayama and Hazel Rose Markus, eds. Pp. 133–196. Washington D.C.: American Psychological Association.

Wootton, Anthony

1976 *Dilemmas of Discourse: Controversies about the Sociological Interpretation of Language.* New York: Holmes and Meier.

Wu, David Y. H.

1982 Psychotherapy and Emotion in Traditional Chinese Medicine. In *Cultural Conceptions of Mental Health and Therapy.* A. Marsella and G. White, eds. Pp. 285–302. Boston: Reidel.

Xu, Y. X.

1994 About ICD-10. *Journal of Clinical Psychological Medicine* 4:224–226.

Xu, Jiqun, and Wang Jingzhi, eds.

1983 *Fangji Xue* 方剂学 (Zhongyi formula). Shanghai: Shanghai Kexue Jishu Chubanshe.

Yamamoto, J., E. K. Yeh, F. Loya, P. Slawson, and M. L. Hurwicz

1985 Are American Psychiatric Outpatients More Depressed Than Chinese Outpatients? *American Journal of Psychiatry* 142:1347–1351.

Yan, Yunxiang

1996 *The Flow of Gifts: Reciprocity and Social Networks in a Chinese Village.* Stanford: Stanford University Press.

Yang, Mayfair

1994 *Gifts, Favors, Banquets: The Art of Social Relationships in China.* Ithaca: Cornell University Press.

Yap, P. M.

1974 *Comparative Psychiatry.* Toronto: University of Toronto Press.

Yin, Huihe, and Bona Zhang, eds.

1989 *Zhongyi Jichu Lilun* 中医基础理论 (Zhongyi basic theories). Shanghai: Shanghai Kexue Jishu Chubanshe.

Ying, Yu-wen

1990 Explanatory Models of Major Depression and Implications for Help-Seeking among Immigrant Chinese-American Woman. *Culture, Medicine and Psychiatry* 14:393–408.

You, Haili

1995a   Defining Rhythm: Aspects of an Anthropology of Rhythm. *Culture, Medicine and Psychiatry* 18:361–384.

1995b   Rhythm in Chinese Thinking: A Short Question for a Long Tradition. *Culture, Medicine and Psychiatry* 18:463–481.

Young, Allan

1982   Rational Men and the Explanatory Model. *Culture, Medicine and Psychiatry* 6: 21–34.

Young, Derson

1989   Neurasthenia and Related Problems. *Culture, Medicine and Psychiatry* 13:131–138.

Yu, Wei, and Minghui Ren

1997   Crisis and Reform of China's Health Care Insurance System. In *In Search of a Chinese Road towards Modernization*. Jixuan Hu, Zhaohui Hong, and Eleni Stavrou, eds. Pp. 143–166. Lewiston: Edwin Mellen Press.

Zhang, Boyu, Dong Jianhua, and Zhou Zhongying, eds.

1985   *Zhongyi Neike Xue* 中医内科学 (Zhongyi internal medicine). Shanghai: Shanghai Kexue Jishu Chubanshe.

Zhang, Jiebin

1959   [1640] *Jingyue Chuanshu* 景岳全书 (Complete works of Zhang Jingyue). Yuesilou Collection. Shanghai: Shanghai Kexue Jishu Chubanshe.

Zhang, Ming-yuan

1989   The Diagnosis and Phenomenology of Neurasthenia: A Shanghai Study. *Culture, Medicine and Psychiatry*. 13: 147–161.

Zhang, Yanhua

2001   Diagnosing Yu-clinical transformation of distress in the modern ractice of chinese medicine. Presented at The 100th Annual Meeting of AAA. Washington D.C.

2007   Negotiating a path to efficacy in a clinic of chinese medicine. Culture, Medicine and Psychiatry V31:1

Zhao, Jinduo, Zhang Jingren, and Zhang Zhen, eds.

1987   *Zhongyi Zhenghou Zhenduanxue* 中医证候诊断学 (Zhongyi syndrome-pattern diagnostics). Beijing: Renmin Wensheng Chubanshe.

Zhen, Zhiya, and Fu Weikang

1991   *Zhongguo Yixue Shi* 中国医学史 (History of chinese medicine). Beijing: Renmin Weisheng Chubanshe.

Zheng, Yanping, Xu Leyi, and Shen Qijie

1986   Styles of Verbal Expression of Emotional and Physical Experiences: A Study of Depressed Patients and Normal Controls in China. *Culture, Medicine and Psychiatry* 10 (3): 231–244.

Zhong, Tai

1988   Zhuangzi Fawei 庄子法微: Shanghai: Shanghai Giuji Chubanshe.

Zhu, Liangchun

2003   *Bianzheng lunzhi yu bianbing lunzhi xiang jiehe de fujian* 辨证论治与辨病论治
       相结合的肤见 (My humble view on combination of pattern differentiation and
       disease differentiation). http://www.100md.com. September 1.

Zito, Angela

1997   *Of Body and Brush: Grand Sacrifice as Text/Performance in Eighteenth-Century
       China.* Chicago: Chicago University Press.

Zito, Angela, and Tani E. Barlow, eds.

1994   *Body, Subject and Power in China.* Chicago: Chicago University Press.

Index

adjustment, process of, 123, 124. *See also* attuning (*tiao*)

aesthetics, cultural, 14, 30–31, 50

aesthetic values, 30, 42, 44, 51, 58, 139

agitation, 40, 85, 95, 103–104; visceral, 91, 100, 101, 117. See also *zangzao*

Ames, Roger, 26, 51, 148n27, 154n51, 155n2, 156 n22

anger (*nu*), 2, 32, 40, 50, 54–55, 59, 63–64, 66–67, 72–74, 87, 92, 95–98, 103. See also *qiqing*

anxiety, 12, 58, 66, 68, 73, 101, 116, 147n1; as *jiaolu*, 114, 116–117, 166n20; as *you*, 66, 68

attuning (*tiao*), 6, 14, 51, 65, 104–105, 108, 110, 112, 123–125, 136–137, 139–140, 142

bei (grief/sadness), 40, 64, 66, 68, 73, 147n1, 161n55. See also *qiqing*

bentunqi (running pig illness/syndrome), 84–85, 164n44

bianzheng (differentiation of patterns/syndromes), 76, 78, 80–81, 90, 163n35, 167n.24; *bagang* (eight rubrics), 78, 82, 162nn9–10; *bingyin* (illness factor), 78, 79; *liujing* (six patterns), 24, 78, 82. 162n9; *zangfu* (visceral systems), 78, 82. See also *bianzheng lunzhi*

bianzheng lunzhi (differentiating patterns/syndromes and determin-

ing treatment/therapies), 14, 28, 74, 78, 81–83, 107, 109, 144, 163n35, 163n37

bianzheng shizhi. See *bianzheng lunzhi*

Bilmes, Jack, 107, 116

bing, 76, 80–83. *See also* illness

biomedicine, 6, 9, 11, 15, 19, 23, 33, 67, 81, 83, 108, 110, 140, 150n2, 154n46, 165n17; as Western medicine (*xiyi*), 6, 13, 15, 17, 18, 19–22, 29, 75, 82–83, 110, 149n58, 150nn2–3, 151n10, 153 n.31, 163 n.36

bitter mouth, 91, 95, 96, 102, 111

blockage (*du* or *butong*), as Chinese medical symptoms, 32, 44–46, 64, 74, 88–90, 93–94, 97, 110, 118, 119, 122, 125

blood (*xue*), 39, 49, 67, 68, 70, 71, 79, 91, 93, 100–103, 112

body: as embodiment, 2–3, 31, 36; discourse or language of , 5, 14, 35–36; mind-body dichotomy, 6, 8, 31, 33–34. *See also* somatization

body-person or body-self (*shenti*), 3, 8, 14, 31, 35–36, 47, 49–51, 53, 65, 67, 105, 132, 134, 139–142, 157n36

bones (*gu*), 37, 68, 70

boundaries, between Chinese and Western medicines, 17

Brownell, Susan, 2, 36, 155n5, 157n35

CA. *See* conversation analysis

Made in the USA
Las Vegas, NV
24 August 2021